A NEW COMPACT

MARY JANE KORNACKI
with Jack Silversin

A NEW COMPACT

Aligning

PHYSICIAN-ORGANIZATION
EXPECTATIONS

to Transform Patient Care

ACHE Management Series

Health Administration Press
Chicago, Illinois

Your board, staff, or clients may also benefit from this book's insight. For more information on quantity discounts, contact the Health Administration Press Marketing Manager at (312) 424-9470.

Library of Congress Cataloging-in-Publication Data

Kornacki, Mary Jane, author.
  A new compact : aligning physician–organization expectations to transform patient care / Mary Jane Kornacki with Jack Silversin.
     p. ; cm.
  Includes bibliographical references and index.
  ISBN 978-1-56793-703-9 (alk. paper)
  I. Silversin, Jacob B., author. II. Title.
  [DNLM: 1. Health Services Administration. 2. Physician's Role. 3. Contracts. 4. Hospital–Physician Relations. 5. Interprofessional Relations. 6. Organizational Case Studies. 7. Professional Practice—organization & administration. W 62]
  RA971
  362.1068—dc23
                          2014043455

Acquisitions editor: Janet Davis; Project manager: Andrew Baumann; Manuscript editor: Sharon Sofinski; Cover designer: Marisa Jackson; Layout: PerfecType

Found an error or a typo? We want to know! Please e-mail it to hapbooks@ache.org and put "Book Error" in the subject line.

For photocopying and copyright information, please contact Copyright Clearance Center at www.copyright.com or (978) 750-8400.

Health Administration Press
A division of the Foundation of the American
College of Healthcare Executives
One North Franklin Street, Suite 1700
Chicago, IL 60606-3529
(312) 424-2800

Contents

Part I Compact: What It Is and How It Helps

Part II Stories of Compact Development and Implementation

Part III Moving Forward: Lessons and Guides

Physicians have always had an awkward relationship with organizations. From our earliest moments in training, we are told that we bear personal responsibility for our care decisions. We are specifically taught to work independently, not to trust anyone else's history and physical exam, and to make our own judgments about diagnosis and treatment. We don't learn how to work in teams—either with other physicians, or with other professions. And we most certainly do not learn how to partner with administrators and colleagues to improve processes and systems of care. So we come to see ourselves as splendid individual professionals focused heroically on quality. We believe that we achieve results largely because of our own dedication and skills, often despite the efforts of managers, who seem to be focused on costs. We tolerate the organizations in which we find ourselves, as long as they don't get in the way of our work and treat us with appropriate respect.

There have always been a few oddball exceptions, such as military medicine during combat, large multispecialty group practices such as the Mayo Clinic, and some staff-model HMOs. In these organizational settings, physicians recognized that they could be more effective if they worked in partnership with each other, and came to appreciate the value of competent administrators.

Over the last decade, however, these atypical physician–organization relationships have started to become less the exception and more the rule. The majority of physicians now are employed in some sort of hospital or group practice setting. The advent of healthcare reform has accelerated this trend and has spawned new organization forms such as accountable care organizations, with challenging new tasks such as responsibility for the overall costs of care for a population.

The leaders of these new organizations face a fundamentally transformational task. From my perspective, they seem to devote a lot of time and energy to *form*—getting the governance structure right, for example. They also seem to spend great effort on *finances*, making sure the physician compensation system seems fair, equitable, and aligned with external payment models. And they devote considerable technical resources to supporting new *functions,* such as coordination of care.

But, in my view, far too few of the leaders of these new organizations create a fundamentally different *feeling*—specifically, among the physicians who are members, and between those physicians and their administrators and leaders. They cannot possibly implement the massive changes needed without the enthusiastic support and leadership of physicians. As one hospital leader said to me, "All change has to go through 'Doctorland' at some point. And it's a jungle."

If these new organizations are to have any chance of success, physicians and administrators will need to jettison old values and patterns of behavior, and adopt new ones, as they *intentionally* create a new culture. If they don't, to paraphrase an old saw, "Feelings will eat Form, Finances, and Function for lunch."

That is why this book is so timely, and so important. It shows the leaders of healthcare organizations why it's necessary to create a new culture. Even better, leaders are shown how to go about that task. It isn't easy. The case studies demonstrate that it takes a lot of time and requires persistent, skilled, adaptive leadership. New cultures can't be copied and pasted; they must be internally grown. Most critical is that the new standards must be embedded in the organization's systems, particularly the human resources systems of recruitment, hiring, promotion, performance feedback, retirement, and, as Edgar Schein so aptly puts it, "excommunication."

I cannot imagine how any modern healthcare organization can adapt to a rapidly evolving environment, and succeed in its core mission, without going through the process of creating a new compact. In my view, a new compact is absolutely essential as a platform for transformational change. Leaders who proceed into the new world without one do so at their own peril.

Why should physicians care about compacts? I would suggest to physicians that they read this book with two compacts in mind—organizational and societal. Just as there has always been an implicit organizational compact characterized by autonomy, protection, and entitlement, there has also been a larger compact between our profession and our society, framed similarly. The key element in the societal compact has been autonomy—a privilege of self-regulation granted by society, earned in large part by astonishing science-driven advances in care over the past century, and also by society's perception of our altruistic professionalism. But in the past two or three decades that professional autonomy has been eroded. Why? Because society now knows that, because of our attachment to individual autonomy, we don't use scientific advances very systematically or effectively. And many would argue that society has also begun to perceive doctors as driven less by altruism and more by money.

It would be difficult to develop a new, explicit "compact" between physicians and society, practically speaking. But what if hundreds of organizations went through this painful process and achieved transformational change in real partnership with physicians? And what if, as a result, society started to notice the benefits of safer, more effective, better coordinated, less costly, more patient- and family-centered care? *Is it not possible that physicians might regain some lost professional autonomy at the societal level, by giving up some individual autonomy at the organizational level?*

James L. Reinertsen, MD

Foreword

Healthcare in today's world is a complex system of interdependent parts. Whether we are talking about the *overall political system* with its government agencies, lobbies, unions, insurance companies, malpractice lawyers, and suppliers of equipment and drugs; about a given *regional health delivery system* including hospitals and clinics; or about a given *hospital with its multiple microsystems* through which patients move, we always reach the same discouraging answer: It is horrendously complicated and interdependent. One frequently encounters the view that fixing the system is hopeless because it has so many interdependent players, each of whom is motivated to pursue his or her own economic and vocational interests.

On the other hand, the disturbing statistics about unnecessary hospital-induced infections and medical errors that cause a large number of patient deaths make it essential that we somehow get a grip on this complex system by finding a point of intervention that will begin to make a difference. We've learned from family therapy that the point of intervention is not necessarily the point where the most immediate harm is done. Rather, the point of intervention has to be a part of the system that is accessible to those who want to produce change and is tightly connected to the other parts of the system. If the point of intervention changes, the rest of the system will have to respond and change as well.

Where is that point of intervention in healthcare? *The interaction between doctors and administrators is the key point of intervention if change in the total system is to be accomplished.*

From my perspective, the healthcare system is driven by several occupational cultures that have different assumptions and values. At the governance level we have evolved *medical administrators* who may have come from medicine or nursing but who have acquired an administrative point of view that is inevitably concerned with economics and efficiency. These folks exist at the government, regional, and local hospital levels. The problems of administrators are similar; this leads to a similar set of perceptions and practices that can be thought of as the *administrative culture.*

From the administrators' point of view, doctors pose several problems: They want more autonomy, they are not cost-conscious, and they resist standardization and other efficiency and safety measures, even when those are based on clear evidence that such measures are helpful.

The delivery of healthcare, however, falls primarily to the *physicians, nurses, and various support staff* in clinics and hospitals. By virtue of their training and the similarity of their tasks, they also acquire a common culture. On closer examination, however, this group consists of several distinct subcultures, the most notable of which are the *doctor culture* and the *nursing culture.* Furthermore, while these two cultures are of equal importance to healthcare delivery, they each have a different status within the system. The way healthcare has evolved has given the doctor culture the position of highest status, as manifested in the frequently heard comment that the system is basically designed for the benefit of the doctors. At some level, this elevated status is warranted by the fact that society has charged doctors with the ultimate responsibility for life-and-death decisions and has supported this responsibility by requiring an exceedingly long and demanding education and training period. As anxious patients, we want doctors to have the expertise and sense of responsibility to take good care of us.

From the doctors' point of view, the administrators pose several problems—their cost-cutting, safety, and other efficiency systems not only infringe on doctors' sense of autonomy (which they have been trained to exercise), but the various procedures also require so much administrative work that they interfere with doctors' practice and consequently increase safety problems because they are so time consuming.

As medicine has become more complex and differentiated, these tensions have become increasingly dysfunctional. If administrators and physicians lack the trust to implement needed changes, delivery of healthcare suffers.

For the healthcare system to work better for society, for patient experience and safety to improve, and for costs to be managed, *both* the doctor culture and the administrator culture have to evolve. For this reason, this book is central in showing how such evolution in the physician and administrator cultures has been successfully launched in a variety of healthcare institutions and can be gradually launched elsewhere. By bringing administrators and doctors together to evolve a new compact in the various subsystems such as a given hospital, both the doctors and the administrators evolve new points of view and find new ways of working together for the benefit of the patients and societal health.

Edgar H. Schein

This book is about doctors and administrators who wanted to strengthen trust and alignment in their organizations and applied the idea of "compact" to their own circumstances.

"Compact" is shorthand for reciprocal expectations that are typically unarticulated and assumed. Jack Silversin and I help organizations transform unstated and likely out-of-date expectations into an explicit pact—one that identifies what doctors are entitled to expect of their organization, and what the organization will expect from physician members. Doing this entails hard work and a lot of time in dialogue with organizations' stakeholders; it means *together* shaping and committing to a philosophy to guide everyone's future actions. For most organizations the process involves new insights for leaders, the acknowledgment of some loss for physicians, and—by the end—a deeper partnership between the two groups. For these reasons, "journey" is an apt metaphor for what the people and their organizations have gone through. All were changed by the activities. Their metamorphoses took time—in some cases, more than a year. And although these new compacts are now written, the new culture and the new relationships that they symbolize continue to evolve.

The act of creating this book was itself a journey—for me—and a deeply personal one. Jack and I introduced the compact as a tool for doctors and administrators to clarify mutual expectations, and in some instances to unpack and process perceptions that had become toxic. He and I have worked in tandem on these projects for more than three decades. I've studied, written about, and been fascinated by the theory and practice of leadership and change since we first began. While both of us work directly with clients, we have divided up the work: Jack most often is the motivational speaker and workshop facilitator, and I usually prepare the background work, design the presentations, and generally support our clients' ongoing efforts.

In almost every instance of compact development and implementation you'll be reading about, Jack was on-site to facilitate a retreat or conduct a series of interviews, then meetings. He has been on the road with clients for three decades, logging hundreds of thousands of miles over the years. He has worked with more than a hundred clients and has exceeded the ten thousand hours of practice Malcolm Gladwell popularized as necessary to achieve mastery! Jack has probably run into every possible variation on the theme of "we can't get our doctors to engage with us." He's especially known for his penetrating insights into issues blocking healthy relationships and his ability to get warring factions to sit down face-to-face. Between us, he has done the lion's share of facilitating compact discussions.

When we decided it was important to publish some accounts of successful compact change, it was clear this was going to be my project. Stepping foot into organizations I had not previously visited but knew very well through Jack's descriptions deepened my own appreciation for the tasks leaders undertook when they committed to compact work. These visits were inspiring and illuminating. I heard poignant stories of pivotal exchanges between meeting participants—some had taken place years earlier but were so salient and resonant that they were recounted as if they had just happened. My visits to these six organizations were not just trips back in time but journeys of deeper understanding about the real usefulness of the construct and the value of what we have spent so many years doing.

The first-person voice when it appears in the narratives is mine. "We" refers to Jack and me. But the thinking and planning behind the compact work as well as the "doing"—advising leaders and facilitating conversations—has been our joint work. The ideas and guidance offered in this book represent us both.

Mary Jane Kornacki

Acknowledgments

Shakespeare's rascal knight, Falstaff, believed that words are but "air." And until committed to paper, they are just that.

A few of these compact stories mention the imperative of finding the "right words" and note that conversations became boisterous as people debated which few words would convey complex ideas. I believe an important part of the process of creating a compact is hashing out which words to include and what each word will mean. This process of wrestling with words brings parties into closer alignment with each other.

For many years, Jack Silversin and I spoke with a wide variety of groups about physician–organization compacts, advising and supporting clients to develop reciprocal agreements. But we hadn't really published much on the topic. As any author can tell you, talking is easy; expressing ideas in writing precisely and clearly—not so much. Getting these words about compacts from air onto the page was a labor in which many people played a part.

First and always, I acknowledge Jack Silversin, my partner in all things. Simply put, without his work with clients on rewriting compacts, there would be no reason for a book. He has been an engaged student of relationships inside healthcare organizations and a tireless advocate of building partnerships and working collaboratively. He has brought the message "we are better together" to audiences across the United States, the United Kingdom, Canada, and the Netherlands for three decades. He has worked with passion to help individuals inside organizations to be better together—by moving beyond recriminations and suspicion and taking up the work of trust building and commitment keeping. To this specific project—in addition to his work with the featured institutions—Jack has contributed the chapter devoted to questions from the field, adding his voice and insights; has provided thoughtful advice for many chapters; and was my sounding board throughout.

Edgar Schein has been both friend and mentor, and I am ever so grateful for all his encouragement and guidance through the years. His investment as an early reader of drafts of this book and his spot-on critiques, insights, and feedback have made it far better. His foreword puts into clear prose why the focus on physician–administrator relationships is so critical to any forward progress in this industry. My debt to Ed extends well beyond this book, however. As a pioneer in organizational development and an early investigator of psychological contracts in the workplace, his are the shoulders I, and Jack, humbly stand on.

This is a book of case histories only because a group of executives and senior leaders responded positively to our request to look closely at what they had done and provide for the wider health administration community an unflinching look at what compact work actually involves. I offer special thanks to those who welcomed the opportunity to participate and provided open access to their organizations. Included are Drs. Andy Dorwart, Keith Fernandez, Charles Hipp, David Holloway, Gregory Long, Larry Morrissey, Peggy Naleppa, Tom Riccio, and Steve Scallon as well as Barbara Gunder and Susan Wright.

Dr. Gary Kaplan did more than open the doors of his organization (Virginia Mason) for this project. Over the years he has been an indispensible thought partner and co-creator, along with Jack, of talks and presentations that feature the role a compact can play in care delivery transformation. He has been a staunch supporter of our work, but above all, his friendship over many years has been a most special gift.

As Virginia Mason board members, Carolyn Corvi and Jamie Orlikoff went above and beyond any formal duties and took the time necessary to ensure that the story of their board's compact was accurately related.

Kathy Franklin was officially retired at the time of my visit to Appleton, Wisconsin, to learn about ThedaCare's compact experience, but she was a full collaborator, giving me not only the historical perspective but also her well-trained organizational-development insights on the process and its results. My thanks to Kathy for reading drafts of the ThedaCare case and providing critiques.

In the course of this project, I interviewed dozens of physicians, managers, executives, nurses, and other staff in the organizations featured. I am grateful to each person for generously giving their time and trust. Just about every organization put a miracle worker at my disposal—an executive assistant who set up my schedule and squeezed doctors into what were often brief on-site visits. Special thanks for such miracles to Karen Long, Rita Middleton, Gloria Muneton, Sharon Roberts, and Isabelle Ryan.

One of the joys of our work is meeting and getting to know individuals with extraordinary leadership talent. Jack and I are both honored to call Dr. Michael Shabot a friend and collaborator. On first meeting Michael at Cedars-Sinai Medical Center (Los Angeles), Jack knew he was working with an exceptional physician who deeply understood the power of internal hospital relationships to affect patient care. I thank him for the hours he gave this project, explaining the intricacies of clinical integration and how Memorial Hermann Physician Network successfully uses its compact to engage independent doctors.

Jim Reinertsen's contributions to care improvement and physician leadership are widely known and respected. Both Jack and I offer appreciation for the comments in his foreword. Thirty years ago we were newcomers to healthcare consulting. Jim's writings about physician autonomy gave credence to our conclusions, giving us more courage to call it out as an impediment to organizational transformation and care improvement.

I am deeply indebted to my friend, colleague, and editor, Leslie Cohen, who always found the right word and rendered my drafts coherent and readable. Her unfailing support, her belief in this project, and her dedication to doing what it took to meet deadlines made the work of producing this book all the easier.

At Health Administration Press, Janet Davis was my champion. Her experience and wisdom are appreciated, as were her patience and unflagging support at every stage of this project.

Friend Stacia Talberth is the kind of reader every author needs. Her attention to detail helped enormously in the final preparation of this manuscript.

Jack and I have been blessed to have spent our professional careers in the health-care arena. To the multitude of doctors and executives whom we've had the privilege to associate with, advise, listen to, and learn from, we owe our deepest thanks. We are both indebted to all of them for trusting us and giving us the opportunity to contribute.

Mary Jane Kornacki

Introduction

"Let's get down to business: What's a physician compact and why should I care?"

Whether you're a healthcare manager, an executive, a trustee, or a physician with—or without—formal leadership responsibility, that's a highly relevant question. Other providers, clinicians, and frontline staff with whom doctors work also have a large stake in the answers to these questions.

The healthcare industry is reeling from seismic shifts in how healthcare services are paid for, how quality and value are defined, and what consumers expect. Complexity is accelerating. Across the developed world, healthcare reform is a priority. Government initiatives and market forces are driving care to be better, more affordable, more efficient, and safer. All this translates into a mandate for executives to bring change to their organizations.

Jack Silversin and I are principals of a healthcare consulting firm that has helped organizations in the United States, United Kingdom, and Canada create explicit physician–organization compacts that support the vision these organizations want to achieve. Clients include group practices, hospitals, academic medical centers, and systems.

Many of the more popular strategies to respond to the pressures for reform are largely untested, and the likelihood of their success isn't all that clear. Will consolidations and mergers save money or ultimately raise costs? Is employing physicians a practical way to capture patients and ensure physician cooperation? Does penalizing hospitals for poor quality reduce costs more efficiently than incenting physicians for complying with known best practices? Can hospitals and independent medical groups compete for ancillary care and diagnostics and still collaborate in care delivery? Will team-based medical care increase primary care capacity?

Regardless of which strategies a board endorses and executives pursue, *the difference between success and failure is physician engagement*. Passive acquiescence will kill a change initiative. Physicians *must* actively support and participate in measures to improve care, reduce waste, coordinate treatment plans with colleagues, and make efficient use of available resources. Physicians are the linchpins of reform. The 2010 Affordable Care Act emphasizes care coordination and is a case in point: Without changed physician behavior, efficiencies are not likely to be realized. By withholding support, physicians can derail a merger, scuttle a safety improvement initiative, or sabotage any policy that relies on their cooperation. To gain that support and engagement, they need a new compact—a new agreement between doctors and administrators as to what each should give and expect in return.

In this book, I present the case histories of a number of healthcare organizations we have worked with that have successfully intervened to construct a new compact with physicians through dialogue and respectful airing of different perspectives. My intention is to offer a deep dive into the psychological contract—long-held, unarticulated expectations—that exists between physicians and healthcare organizations. These expectations thwart reform; they must be openly renegotiated to better support the changes your organization needs to deliver affordable, quality care.

AUTONOMY, PROTECTION, ENTITLEMENT

When we first began to consult to healthcare organizations in the early 1980s, Jack and I were puzzled by some of what we saw and experienced. "Why would physicians do that?" we wondered more than once. Why would physicians, clearly aware of a colleague's brusque manner with patients and its impact on the reputation of the whole group, hesitate to call out such behavior? Why would partners resist changing physician-centric policies that cause them to lose market share to competitors? How is it that, when shown clear and compelling evidence of performance or quality shortfalls, many would rather niggle over the validity of data than brainstorm ideas for improvement?

We began to appreciate the complexity of physicians' relationships with their organizations. One thing we observed early on was that a majority of group-practice doctors enjoyed the best of all possible worlds: the benefits of close proximity to colleagues, some measure of safety in numbers, and, by mutual consent, the privileges of solo practice—getting to do things their own way. The golden rule of medical group practice could be summed up as: "We're all great doctors here, so I won't tell you how to practice and trust that you won't tell me how to, either."

That's a great deal for a professional, but for organizations that want to innovate, it has been a liability for some time. During retreats that Jack and I facilitated, we often asked physicians to list the privileges they enjoy as part of the practice and the obligations they owe the practice. Invariably, the list of privileges was far longer. Some groups of physicians struggled with whether they have *any* obligations to the larger organization (as opposed to patients), if that term is defined as "must do or be terminated." After much debate, one group agreed that staying out of legal trouble was the only line that, if crossed, would lead to separation from the practice.

After conducting this exercise with numerous clients, we've boiled down what we hear most doctors feel is their due: *autonomy, protection,* and *entitlement.* Physicians do not create these expectations from thin air; these outlooks are constructed in medical school days when professional identity is developing. And, in most organizations, they are reinforced during the recruitment process and in daily interactions with other physicians, staff, managers, and even board members. Such expectations are profoundly related to the compact we as a society have with the medical profession. As healers and holders of privileged information, physicians since Hippocrates have enjoyed elevated status. Until recent pressure for healthcare change gathered unstoppable momentum, this "old compact" supported the success of medical groups, community hospitals, and academic medical centers by allowing them to attract and retain good physicians.

ORIGINS OF THE PSYCHOLOGICAL CONTRACT

In our work, we use the terms "psychological contract" and "compact" more or less interchangeably. As noted above, a psychological contract is a set of unarticulated expectations, a mental construct. "Compact" means essentially the same—the terms not of a legal contract so much as of the relationship between an employer and employee (Goman 1997). However, unlike psychological contracts, some compacts are explicit and written.

In its original conceptualization, the psychological contract referred to an exchange between employer and employee. Chris Argyris (1960) is credited with first applying the notion of "implicit reciprocal agreements" to the workplace. Drawing on his study of the work relationships in a manufacturing plant, he used "psychological work contracts" to refer to implicit agreements between employees and their foremen. Among his conclusions is that "the employee will maintain high production, low grievances, etc., if the foremen guarantee and respect the norms of the employee informal culture (i.e., let the employees alone, make certain they make adequate wages and have secure jobs)" (Argyris 1960, 97).

According to Edgar Schein (1980, 22), an early investigator of this construct, "the notion of a psychological contract implies that there is an unwritten set of expectations operating at all times between every member of an organization and the various managers and others in that organization." Schein considers employee expectations to be "such things as salary or pay rate, working hours, benefits and privileges that go with a job, guarantees not to be fired unexpectedly, and so on. Many of these expectations are implicit and involve the person's sense of dignity and worth." The organization, for its part, has tacit expectations of those it pays and counts on to carry out its business, including expectations "that the employee will enhance the image of the organization, will be loyal, will keep organizational secrets, and will do his or her best on behalf of the organization (that is, will always be highly motivated and willing to make sacrifices for the organization)" (Schein 1980, 23).

W. H. Whyte, Jr., in *The Organization Man* (2002, 129), summed up a 1950s-era compact when he wrote: "Be loyal to the company and the company will be loyal to you." Workers put in an honest day's effort in exchange for pay and a range of other benefits such as health insurance (after World War II), cost-of-living raises, and some retirement or pension allotment. Loyalty in exchange for job security "worked" for employees and for the firms that hired them. The employer could count on a stable workforce with predictable, fixed costs, and employees could expect to have a long-term job.

COMPACTS CHANGE AS NEEDS CHANGE

Today, a "loyalty for job security" psychological contract, with its paternalistic undertones, strikes us as out of date. It is an unwritten set of expectations from an earlier era—one in which the workforce was predominantly male, large employers were primarily manufacturers, and management was not just top-down but command and control. Such a compact supported business success when predictability and stability were critical to fulfilling an organization's mission.

Jack Welch, former General Electric (GE) chairman and CEO, summed up a compact change that was foundational to GE's transformation: "We had an implicit psychological contract based on perceived lifetime employment. . . . This produced a paternal, feudal, fuzzy kind of loyalty. . . . The new psychological contract is that jobs at GE are the best in the world for people willing to compete" (quoted in Tichy and Charan 1989, 120).

Hoffman, Casnocha, and Yeh (2013), in the *Harvard Business Review*, discuss the need for explicit compacts that reflect the requirements of twenty-first-century employers and employees. The solutions they offer reveal the demise of the lifetime-employment compact as well as the shortcomings of an every-man-for-himself alternative. In their view, a new-world compact especially relevant to high-tech start-ups could be summarized as: "Employees invest in the company's adaptability; the company invests in employees' employability" (51).

Today, multiple pressures in the healthcare world are eroding the traditional physician social contract and taking a toll on physician morale. A fundamental shift is occurring in decades-old, unspoken expectations, recalibrating the relationships between doctor and patient and between doctor and organization, and greatly undermining professional satisfaction (Edwards, Kornacki, and Silversin 2002). Most wrenching for physicians is having been socialized during their training with certain expectations only to find that the "deal" has changed in ways that are, in their eyes, less advantageous—all without conversation or even acknowledgment that such has happened. This erosion of the old, assumed deal is one source of physicians' growing disillusionment and frustration.

INTERVENTION

Recently, I've seen evidence that the newer generation of physicians is beginning to hold different assumptions than their older colleagues, especially about professional autonomy and the need to be an active participant in quality improvement, including standardization of care processes. One young physician told me she was "beyond surprised" to learn there was no standard tray setup in her outpatient clinic. She could only conclude that her work would be rife with inefficiencies if staff were still tailoring trays to doctors' individual preferences. Young physicians tend to have different expectations regarding work–life balance, show a marked proclivity toward specialties where they can work "by the clock," and gravitate toward employment instead of independence or partnership. Many trained under work-hour rules that were more restrictive than those applicable to earlier generations of doctors.

Important to keep in mind, however, is that this newer generation is still being socialized by those for whom autonomy, protection, and entitlement were (and in many cases still are) the holy grail. Thus, even though older doctors are aging out of practice and out of teaching in medical schools, the evolutionary path to a more adaptive compact is dishearteningly slow.

For this reason, given the quality, safety, and economic imperatives for change, we must intervene to accelerate the successful adoption of an urgently needed new compact. The phrase "facilitated adaptation"—used by geneticists who manipulate genes for a specific purpose (Rich 2014)—is a fitting descriptor for the process of negotiating new, reciprocal commitments. *Compact work is an intentional act that helps move along an evolutionary process already underway.* It puts physicians and their organizations on a better footing to respond to current imperatives and builds capability to respond to changes just over the horizon.

OVERVIEW OF THE BOOK

Chapter 1 draws a direct line between the traditional physician compact and physicians' slow response to the imperatives organizations face. The case is made for open renegotiation of a more functional physician–organization compact.

Chapter 2 summarizes steps in a compact development and implementation process that our clients have found helpful. This overview of how compact change can happen is a guide to the stages traveled by the organizations in the cases that follow.

I visited six different communities and interviewed numerous change participants to hear firsthand how their compact work changed relationships and furthered organizational success. Their stories are presented in Part II, Chapters 3–9.

The organizations range from a four thousand–member physician association that is a part of the nine-hospital Memorial Hermann Health System to a group practice of fifty providers in Stillwater, Minnesota. The story of Virginia Mason Medical Center's compact journey, which started in 2001, and its connection to its ground-breaking Virginia Mason Production System is included. ThedaCare in Appleton, Wisconsin, sought to expand its system by acquiring primary care practices in the mid-1990s. It undertook a compact process with those physicians to strengthen systemness and to create a brand recognized for outstanding quality. Two stories focus on compacts at community hospitals staffed by employed, independent, and contracted physicians: Salem Hospital and Peninsula Regional Medical Center. The final chapter of this part of the book is based on an interview with a seasoned executive who worked in both the English National Health Service and the Department of Health and applied the concept of clear, reciprocal expectations to build strong partnerships with leaders of other organizations.

Following these case histories, in Part III the focus shifts to lessons and their applications. Chapter 10 summarizes insights and lessons from across these organizations. Chapter 11 offers a planning tool (built from the steps outlined in Chapter 2) with prompts and questions to guide a compact process your organization might undertake. Chapter 12, in question-and-answer format, provides practical advice from Jack Silversin, who was directly involved in the featured cases. I have included, at the end of the book, a list of suggested readings that you will find helpful if you decide to pursue this work.

◆ ◆ ◆

As you will realize in reading these cases, compacts aren't inherently good or bad. There is no "best" compact. At issue is the match between the largely unspoken expectations your physicians carry and the strategies your organization must pursue now to thrive tomorrow. This book will help you clarify whether your current physician–organization compact is as supportive of the organization's aims as it needs to be—and if outdated expectations are a barrier to change, how that compact can be re-created.

Chris Argyris (1977) wrote a good deal about learning organizations, the subject of Peter Senge's classic book, *The Fifth Discipline* (1990). By learning together how to become better partners and more change resilient, the doctors and administrators in the stories that follow demonstrate that it is possible to address some of the dysfunctions that thwart change and allow unconstructive relationships to persist. They not only share the details of their compact journey but also illustrate the spirit of looking below the surface that is the hallmark of what Argyris and Senge both noted as a learning organization.

Part I

COMPACT: WHAT IT IS AND HOW IT HELPS

CHAPTER 1

What Is a Compact—and Why Is a New One Needed?

Here are just a few troubling situations in which executives and physicians have found themselves that suggest a new relationship is needed:

- When they signed on, physicians acquired by an expanding healthcare system were promised they would generally be left alone. However, angered by reports showing they're not sending their referrals to the system's employed specialists and by the healthcare system's demands that they standardize supplies and justify the hiring of support staff, the physicians claim they are victims of a bait and switch. The icing on the cake, as they see it, is the news that they are to take on the system's name—and give up their own—as part of a branding strategy.
- Due diligence prevents the hospital's CEO from discussing with physicians the details of a potential merger that was reported in the local newspaper. Independent doctors in the community interpret the lack of up-front communication as indicating the CEO intends to "sell them down the river" and sign an affiliation agreement with an integrated system that employs its physicians.
- Doctors who halfheartedly bought into Lean principles are discouraged from further engagement in the improvement philosophy because of "top-down tactics" calling for guidelines developed at another site to be introduced at their site. They see this action as going against their tradition of distributed leadership. Believing the administration is playing hardball, the physicians reject the applicability of guidelines not invented at their site instead of trying to tailor the guidelines to their local conditions.
- Administrators see greed and the desire for control as the motives behind a local nonemployed neurology group's decision to build its own sleep medicine

center. The neurologists see the center as necessary for their survival as market conditions shift because it will allow them to remain independent for as long as possible and strengthen their position if they need to integrate with a larger enterprise.

The disconnect between managers and doctors is not exactly news. Much has been written on the divergent worldviews, training, roles and responsibilities, and values orientation of managers and doctors. The dysfunction in this relationship and the consequences of that dysfunction have long been of interest to both academics and practitioners (Davies and Harrison 2003; Degeling et al. 2003; Garelick and Fagin 2005). Amer Kaissi (2005), a professor of healthcare administration, has examined the underlying factors in this relationship from several different perspectives. He concludes that managers and physicians represent different tribes as a result of cultural differences. Nigel Edwards and colleagues (2003, 609), introducing a themed issue of the *British Medical Journal* on doctors and managers, state, "The fundamental problem is a paradox between calls for a common set of values and the need to recognise that doctors and managers do and should think differently."

Empirical research and theoretical models aren't needed to make the point that increasing pressure and uncertainty about the future usually chip away at trust and partnership. Instead of serving as catalysts for meaningful doctor–manager partnerships and for obtaining solid trustee support, the trends and pressures now operating to reform healthcare (Chassin 2013; Cutler and Morton 2013; Jost 2014; Moses et al. 2013) have usually instigated anger, insecurity, and misunderstanding between concerned and well-intentioned individuals. We know from our work that such problems can in fact *unite* these parties—so why do they lead to such division and resentment in many institutions?

THE TRADITIONAL
PHYSICIAN–ORGANIZATION COMPACT

One important reason for the tension between physicians and managers is the implicit compact, or psychological contract, that binds both parties—a compact that has gone unchallenged for a long time. The traditional compact is a major source of slow change, failed attempts at change, and strained relationships.

Denise Rousseau has written extensively about psychological contracts in a variety of organizations. She and her colleague Martin Greller offer the following definition, which I have annotated to explore this concept in relation to physicians:

The psychological contract encompasses the actions employees [physicians] believe are expected of them and what response they expect in return from their employer [the organization in which they practice medicine—be they employed, contracted, or independent]. (Rousseau and Greller 1994, 386)

When physicians are asked to make a change—for example, to follow a treatment protocol, input orders via computer, or practice team-based care—and they push back with the comment "I didn't come here for that," they are expressing their reality. As far as many doctors are concerned, veering off preferred routines or established patterns at the behest of others isn't part of the unspoken deal—the traditional, implicit compact—they agreed to when they became physicians, nor is it, in their eyes, an obligation of organizational citizenship. Even when physician leaders request the change, physicians can feel their inherent sense of medical professionalism—and the implicit deal—have been violated. The traditional compact between physicians and organizations looks similar to the one represented in Exhibit 1.1.

The pact that physicians feel is—or should be—operating isn't a figment of their imagination. It's rooted in centuries-old traditions and in their training; it's reinforced by everyday interactions and by the enticements organizations offer to recruit talent. Administration colludes with physicians in many ways to keep elements of the old compact intact. Is the typical hiring discussion designed to entice doctors by offering them what they want and expect to hear? Or does the organization lay out a deal reflecting what behaviors it expects from physicians and what, in turn, physicians are entitled to expect? Does the administration accept antisocial behavior from talented physicians to keep them from taking their business elsewhere?

Exhibit 1.1 Traditional Physician–Organization Compact

Physician Responsibilities (Physician "Gives")	Organization Responsibilities (Physician "Gets")
◆ Treat patients. ◆ Provide quality care—as you define it.	◆ Respect physicians' clinical autonomy. ◆ Protect physicians from the business side of the enterprise, from market forces, and from change. ◆ Allow entitlements commensurate with physicians' status (including not holding them accountable in the way that other staff are) and treat them as key customers.

Or does it make clear that respectful behavior is an expectation of all doctors and administrators?

In short, if expectations are left unsaid in the early days of joining the organization, each doctor will subjectively interpret what he or she owes the organization. If conscious attention is not paid to matching physicians' expectations with the organization's, physicians will by default carry forward unconscious legacy expectations of autonomy, protection, and entitlement.

A Barrier to Needed Change

The traditional physician compact (Exhibit 1.1) is a barrier to engaging doctors in changes that organizations need to implement. When asked to take on responsibilities outside of the implied compact, physicians feel angry or frustrated and are labeled "uncooperative," which unleashes a cascade of unhelpful interactions. If relationships between doctors and the administration and trustees are in disrepair, the stress brought on by new imperatives intensifies this harmful dynamic. The result is a deepening frustration on all sides.

As noted earlier, as credentialed professionals most physicians harbor certain expectations of the "workplace" in which they see patients. These expectations do not vary by employment status or organizational setting—or even national boundaries. What most physicians expect to give is medical care—the best they can. Until recently, good care has been largely determined by "what works in my clinical experience," locally accepted practices, knowledge gained at professional events, insurance reimbursement, and journal reports of clinical research. In exchange for providing care, doctors tacitly expect respect for their clinical autonomy; protection from changes, market forces, and worries about the cost of care; and entitlements commensurate with their status (e.g., tolerance for behavior unacceptable in other staff, reserved parking).

The way that the unspoken compact bollixes attempts to introduce change becomes clear if one views autonomy, protection, and entitlement alongside typical challenges most healthcare organizations face today. The two columns in Exhibit 1.2 illustrate the mismatch between physicians' expectations and challenges that must be addressed.

If you customize the right-hand column of Exhibit 1.2 to your institution, you'll likely find at least some mismatch between doctors' expectations and what your organization needs from them. When they see the lists side by side, many doctors recognize the lack of synchrony as the source of their internal dissonance and

Exhibit 1.2 Mismatch of Physician Expectations and Organizational Imperatives

Physicians' Tacit Expectations (Legacy Compact)	Typical Challenges Healthcare Organizations Face
◆ Autonomy ◆ Protection ◆ Entitlement	◆ Coordinate care across intra- and interorganizational boundaries ◆ Reduce cost ◆ Eliminate waste ◆ Practice evidence-based medicine, follow protocols ◆ Implement electronic medical records ◆ Move care to less expensive setting

say, "Now I know why I feel the way I do." To the extent this old compact exists, responding to any imperatives is slow and difficult.

Operating on Parallel Tracks No Longer Works

Imagine two railroad tracks running parallel to each other. One represents the board's and management's work: visioning, strategizing, organizing, and executing plans. The other represents the physician's work: patient care and, in some institutions, research and teaching. This two-track approach worked well for healthcare organizations for decades. The traditional compact allowed physicians to ignore finances, strategy, and personnel management and represented no real barrier to institutional success.

Today, such a two-track orthodoxy greatly undermines the organization's capacity for change. Physicians need to understand, at some basic level, how their actions affect economic performance and patient satisfaction, which is increasingly linked to reimbursement. If rank-and-file physicians are exempt from having business literacy, they cannot constructively dialogue about needed change. With little understanding of the broader context, physicians see administrators as "the heavies" when they ask the physicians to behave differently. Instead of collectively working to make continued success more likely, physicians direct their energy toward questioning the need for change.

At the same time, clinical implications attach to almost every decision an administrator makes—thus, administrators must listen closely when physicians question their edicts. How well does each party understand the other's imperatives? A process to define new mutual commitments, to co-develop an explicit compact, helps both doctors and administrators expand their understanding of life "on the other track."

A NEW COMPACT MEANS ADAPTIVE CHANGE

The organizations whose compact journeys you will read about in this book all approached the work as the *adaptive change* it is. Here are two key points about adaptive change relevant to compact work:

1. At the start of a process no predefined solution exists; one has to be created.
2. Those who will be implementing the remedy have to be among those who figure it out.

The term "adaptive change" has been popularized by Ronald Heifetz and his colleagues at Harvard's Kennedy School of Government (Heifetz 1998; Heifetz and Laurie 1997; Heifetz and Linsky 2002a, 2002b; Heifetz, Linsky, and Grashow 2009). They distinguish adaptive change from what they call "technical change," in which the problem is well defined and a solution exists. Even if you don't know the best solution to a technical problem, someone else does. Meeting a technical challenge doesn't call for anyone to abandon cherished traditions or personal values. Flat tires are fixed, bones are set, injections are given, and diuretics are swallowed—without angst or tension.

But adaptive changes do increase anxiety and stress; for that reason, we would rather avoid them. Typically, such changes evoke loss because they mean giving up a practice that has worked well or a long-held belief. Merging with another entity, reporting to a new department head, and becoming more transparent in reporting errors represent adaptive changes.

Asking physicians to give up or modify deeply held assumptions that are tightly bound to their sense of professionalism is asking them to undergo a profound adaptive change. That process takes a good deal of conversation, venting, and even grieving along the way. If the process to define a new compact resembles a checklist exercise or stifles real conversation, it won't result in meaningful compact change.

REPLACE AN AMBIGUOUS, UNARTICULATED COMPACT WITH AN EXPLICIT ONE

Given the strained physician–administrator relationships and demands for change, it may seem an awkward time to discuss something as seemingly ethereal as a "new compact." However, such discussion is the prescription for easing some of the burden of mistrust and anger and for building resilience in these critical relationships. At this juncture a new compact—one that aligns physicians' expectations with administrators' views—is crucial.

What would a new compact look like?

◆ *First, a new compact would be explicit and written.* It would identify reciprocal expectations—what physicians are entitled to expect of their organization and what the organization is entitled to expect of them.

◆ *Second, the compact would be linked to the organization's vision.* Administrators and physicians share that vision. At the start, doctors and administrators have to agree that they're going someplace together. This definition of the future state will be different for each organization. To enable reasoned discussion about a desired future state, administrators may need to present facts and figures to physicians and help them understand what they mean. Without business literacy that allows physicians to translate market conditions into likely financial impact, their views about what is possible for the institution's future may be unrealistic.

◆ *Third, compact change would be recognized for being the adaptive change that it is.* Because developing new expectations involves adjustments to deeply held assumptions and beliefs, the direct involvement of physicians, executives, and administrative leaders is needed. Adopting a compact developed elsewhere, tweaking it in an executive meeting, and announcing, "Here's our new compact" will only generate cynicism. Everyone who will be required to meet the compact's expectations must have some voice in what is proposed.

◆ ◆ ◆

The implicit compact in your institution may already be eroding from the demands that your organization makes of physicians. If physicians' unarticulated expectations are whittled away—or dashed—and no meaningful substitute is offered, it's little wonder many physicians feel let down or betrayed. Erasing bits of their old compact without any conversation or substitution for cherished traditions doesn't serve anyone well; unhappy doctors are not the most compassionate healers or the most engaged partners to implement strategy or innovate solutions to organizational challenges.

As the cases in this book make clear, the challenge ahead for you and your institution is to identify physicians' and administrators' expectations and disappointments, face them, and help the parties move forward together to build a compact that is a solid foundation for change.

CHAPTER 2

A Template for Compact Change

In 1995, the idea of developing an explicit compact between doctors and their organization was brand new, one that Jack Silversin presented at a meeting for group practice leaders. In the following years he presented numerous times on this topic at American Medical Group Association conferences and Institute for Healthcare Improvement meetings.

The first clients to dip their toes in these waters were innovative medical groups. In 2001, the medical staff at Cedars-Sinai Medical Center in Los Angeles led a compact development process with Silversin's guidance. Other organizations did compact work as early as 2000–2003; these organizations tended to identify themselves as early adopters of new ideas.

Many saw connections between the quality-improvement movement and the compact, and they clearly recognized that the slow uptake of this important work to make care better and safer was in large part rooted in physician autonomy. Compact dialogue was seen as one way to address the third-rail issue of physician accountability.

The innovative medical groups found that a new, explicit compact was effective in deepening trust and helping direct physicians and administrators toward shared aims. They also found that the compact process takes time and heartfelt commitment.

A SYSTEMATIC PROCESS AUGMENTED
WITH JUDGMENT AND FLEXIBILITY

No lockstep process guarantees success in developing an effective physician–organization compact. For clarity, however, this chapter provides a map of the typical route taken in the cases presented in this book. Chapter 11 expands on the discussion of this typical route, offering a guide for you and others in your organization to consider and plan compact work in your organization.

Essential to compact work are leaders who are able to make judgments about organizational readiness, timing, the degree to which doctors share the organization's vision, and individuals' willingness to own their share of responsibility for the current dynamic. One cannot overstate the importance of good judgment about when it's time—or not—to move on to the next phase of the work.

The following sections briefly describe a sequence of compact work that allows for flexibility along the way.

Bring the Idea Inside and Share It with Others

Although the idea of writing a new compact has gained traction, it isn't well known to many working in healthcare. The first step in a compact process arises naturally when someone reads or hears about the compact, senses its usefulness in solving some problem their organization faces, and shares that awareness with others.

Name the Problem

The second step generally is taken when someone names a challenge the organization needs to solve right away. Change happens only when people feel the pinch of urgency compelling them to move beyond the status quo.

Naming the problem sharpens the sense of urgency. Physician or administrative leaders with the capability and status to begin a change process must have a clear sense of the problem they are seeking to address—and they must grasp how the old, implicit compact impedes the remedy. The problem could be lagging financial performance, an unacceptable patient safety record, or growing physician disenchantment.

Whatever the problem is, it needs to be clearly called out, and the connection between the slow progress in addressing it and the old compact needs to be made. Given the time and resources required to do this work well, leaders must ensure an explicit new compact is an appropriate solution to the problem.

Constitute a Core Working Group

Once clarity about the problem exists, the next step is to constitute a core working group to lead and organize the compact work and address issues such as whose expertise is needed to help with the process, who will help with logistics, and who will be foot soldiers or champions.

This core group is usually pulled together to vet the idea, build support for doing the work, and take the first steps in drafting a new compact. The group typically includes leaders high enough up the hierarchy for their involvement to signal that this work is a priority. Depending on the size of the organization, managers or staff from human resources or the medical staff office can be called to help plan and coordinate meetings.

Given all these tasks, the core working group meets frequently. Their contributions are enriched when they use time between meetings to look for and take note of how the current compact manifests itself in daily life. Tuning in and then sharing observations with others during the core group meetings takes the compact out of the realm of the theoretical and helps the core group deeply appreciate the challenges and benefits of compact change.

Visualize a Different Future

Clarify and Agree on a Shared Vision

If urgency gets our attention, a compelling picture of a better future pushes us forward and sustains us. The compact itself spells out what we expect of each other, but first comes the context—the vision: About *what* exactly do we have expectations of each other? What are we working toward together?

The core group can take the lead on defining this different and better future. Defining the vision might require its own process, one involving input from stakeholders. Or, the core group could draft a statement to be vetted along with a draft compact. The key is that the shared vision (or vision statement) *sets the context* for the compact. It describes a future that all parties can endorse. It must be compelling enough to move people beyond their individual notions of what the future should look like. It must also have practical use beyond public relations.

As part of this process, sharing financial, safety, and other performance-related data as well as national and local trends with physicians is important so that their input will be informed by practical concerns. If they lack basic business literacy, their vision of the future may be a fantasy. Depending on the circumstances, a process to educate physician leaders and physicians about the economic reality and impact of reform may need to take place prior to any vision work if they are to contribute meaningfully.

The investment that organizations need to make to develop enough shared vision to move on to compact work will vary. In some organizations, general consensus on the future direction and the crafting of a preamble for a compact might be all that are needed to specify what all parties are committed to achieving. In such cases, the affirmation of an existing vision can be part of the compact development process. Other organizations might need to engage in a more complex and protracted process to bring together disparate views and develop a shared vision prior to beginning compact work.

Draft a New Compact

Once the core group can articulate where it is heading, it then considers what physicians and the organization need to do to get everyone there. In brief, it drafts a reciprocal code of behaviors that support the shared vision. Some acknowledgment of the current compact—written or implied—is useful to draw a clear distinction between it and the proposed new one.

Viewing the draft as a straw dog (a simple proposal intended to generate comment) is helpful. The core group—or an expanded group doing the drafting—has the task of putting in writing the "gives" and "gets" that others can respond to. Circulating any document produced at this stage as anything other than a conversation starter is not the most effective way to proceed in most instances. Offering a draft compact can kick-start conversation, but if the original drafters are too committed to their own ideas, the engagement process will feel false to those asked to give input.

Engage in Dialogue and Compact Ratification

This step—wide-scale conversation and give-and-take—is the heart of a successful compact process.

The power of the compact lies in these conversations. Genuine engagement may develop through a few general meetings or many departmental meetings. What comprises sufficient discussion is a function of how complex the organization is and how much conversation individuals need to make the transition. The main purpose of these meetings is to talk about imperatives the organization has to respond to and how a compact can help; the purpose is *not* to push the compact through to ratification.

Generally, the straw-dog proposal is presented along with the shared vision as the deep reason for clarifying behaviors. Everyone needs to genuinely appreciate that the current situation is untenable and that a new compact requires new behaviors. Debate, feedback about specific language in the compact and vision statement, and criticisms should all be invited. The key is to keep discussions going until a critical number of medical staff and managers agree that the compact makes sense, they understand the implications for their own behavior, and the mood shifts to "let's move on and implement this!"

Ratification processes vary, but in general the executives, board, or medical executive committee signs off on the compact following whatever process is relevant to adoption of new policy. This final sign-off process usually is not contentious or divisive. In our experience, when the process is well conducted and ample time is devoted to dialogue and give-and-take, the finalization is anticlimactic. Because the big issues have been surfaced and aired, the general feeling is that "everything's been said—let's make it happen."

Implement the Compact

Implementation is how an organization gives the new compact life and "teeth." In this phase, the compact is talked about, used to help make decisions, and integrated into recruiting and hiring practices.

Most important, the compact becomes part of performance conversations. Unless individuals are held accountable under the new compact, its relevance will quickly diminish. Holding people accountable doesn't mean firing those who don't abide by the compact, however. At some point it might come to that, but accountability means first and foremost giving doctors and managers developmental feedback about their behavior. It means noticing and commenting on behavior. There is always a learning curve; when the compact is new, most people will continue their comfortable routines and not automatically demonstrate compact-consistent practices. Leaders need to have the courage and skills to call out discrepancies between agreed-on and actual behavior.

Implementation involves hardwiring the new expectations into policy and procedures. It also means that leaders become more conscious of their power and influence as role models.

Assess and Remediate

If any change is going to be sustained, it has to be tracked and modified. For the compact to become meaningful, mechanisms must exist for honest feedback about the extent to which it is lived. Individuals can get feedback about their behavior through review processes, and leadership can engage in discussion about how well the organization is living up to its commitments.

Leadership might find out early that the compact is making a difference and no changes are needed. But if, after a learning period, the compact seems to have little relevance or people view it with cynicism, leaders should take action to understand why. This last step—assessing and changing as needed—is important if the compact is going to live long enough to become "the way we do things here."

Some organizations find that the wording of their compact created a decade or more ago still serves them well. But part of assessment and remediation includes reexamination of the compact if the organization's desired future state or fundamental purpose is revised. When conditions call for a new vision, it makes sense to revisit the compact to ensure its tenets are still relevant or to identify needed changes. Other opportune times to assess the compact's and vision's goodness of fit are following a merger or when an independent entity becomes part of a larger one. The new organization has to be willing and able to deliver on commitments to physicians or else modify them.

◆ ◆ ◆

As you read the cases that follow, keep in mind that what may appear as a straightforward remedy for alienation between doctors and healthcare organizations is anything but. Compact work isn't about transactions in the usual, legal sense. No one can be faulted for looking at a compact and seeing what looks like legalese, but the compact's language of exchange reflects a *relationship*, not a legal code. Getting to this exchange, in which "you commit to do *this* and we commit to do *that*," involves a good deal of conversation—and a certain amount of vulnerability on both administrators' and physicians' parts. *This relationship-building dimension is a crucial component of the work.* The compact stories in this book illustrate that compacts, at their heart, are about fostering collegiality, which is essential to the executives, managers, physician leaders, and physicians now traversing the unchartered realm of healthcare reform.

Part II

STORIES OF COMPACT DEVELOPMENT AND IMPLEMENTATION

CHAPTER 3

Virginia Mason Medical Center: Compact Supports Transformation of Care

A good deal of well-justified attention has been focused on the transformation of care delivery at Virginia Mason Medical Center (VM) in Seattle, Washington. VM consistently receives high scores on quality measures and in 2011 was named Hospital of the Decade by the Leapfrog Group, which represents large employers across the United States. In a ten-year span this hospital and medical group practice have shaken off a traditional, specialty-oriented reputation to become the acknowledged world leader in applying Toyota Production System Lean tools and management practices to improve healthcare quality and safety. While the great strides VM is making to reduce waste and improve quality get the lion's share of notice, another equally significant transformation has taken place. VM physicians and leadership rewrote the deal that defines what's expected of physicians and what they, in turn, expect from their organization. This new deal underpins strategy and the physicians' embrace of the production system. Seeing VM's achievements and being aware of the direct line between the physician compact and the hospital's transformation brings to mind the Chinese saying: "Those who say it cannot be done should not interrupt the people doing it."

During a tour of VM led by its CEO, Gary Kaplan, MD, I saw firsthand the impact of *kaizen* (a commitment to continuous improvement) and production system tools on space design and care delivery. Experiencing the inpatient orthopedics floor in the new Jones Pavilion is disorienting if you expect the familiar sights and sounds of hospital life. Here, doctors, staff, patients, and architects applied the Lean 3P (production, preparation, process) tools to design a facility that is a testament to innovation and to putting patients and families first. Tranquility reigns; no one appears rushed or frenzied even though every room is full. The screensaver on overhead monitors is the ubiquitous VM strategic plan, visualized as a pyramid with the patient at the apex.

Patient rooms, each with a family zone, circle the periphery and so are flooded with natural light. To maximize patient safety, waste cans are emptied from the outside corridor and patient medications are in a wall unit next to the door of each room. Family or team conference rooms with folding glass doors punctuate the hall. The space is designed for team communication and patient and family well-being. I did not see any centralized nurses' station; instead, pods with two seats and two computers and monitors are strategically placed throughout. Gone are the days when hours were spent "hunting and gathering" needed supplies, information, and so on. Nurses spend the vast majority of their time in face-to-face patient care.

The Jones Pavilion is more than a showcase for whiz-bang, patient-centered design. It's the physical manifestation of the institution's commitment to its Virginia Mason Production System (VMPS). This building reflects innovation and demonstrates the extent to which the institution is in the vanguard of creating new ways to deliver and improve patient care. Here teams of doctors, staff, and patients come together to find and eliminate waste in care processes. Two books chronicle VM's journey to become the preeminent practitioner of Lean in the healthcare field: Charles Kenney's *Transforming Health Care* (2011) and Paul Plsek's *Accelerating Health Care Transformation with Lean and Innovation* (2013).

The leadership at VM—including CEO Kaplan and numerous physician section heads, chairs, and administrative leaders—reported, without reservation, that their physician compact paved the way in enabling Toyota Production System methods to be accepted and then broadly adopted.

In reflecting on the days before undertaking compact work, Kaplan offers the following illustration of life for a new VM doctor:

> The first interactions any newly hired doctor would have with his or her section head and the work unit manager would include the new hire laying out his or her preferences for appointments per day, how long appointments would be, when lunch would be taken. Doctors pretty much designed every aspect of how they would practice, with their own convenience and preferences front and center. In those days, Virginia Mason prided itself on being physician-driven, which boiled down to doctors having ultimate authority. For generations of doctors, at my organization and elsewhere, it was a very sweet deal.

The unspoken deal that allowed doctors to retain authority and autonomy was rarely challenged. Given the stability of psychological contracts, what would disrupt these expectations? For VM doctors, there wasn't one particular day of reckoning, but gradual changes and perceived losses churned up enough angst and doubt to call the old, sweet deal into question.

The year 2000 was an inflection point in VM's history. That year, both changes in market dynamics and longstanding board concerns came more sharply into focus. This confluence of issues started a change process that included a new physician compact.

BACKGROUND

VM was founded in 1920 by physicians who based it on the Mayo Clinic model. They created one organization where patients could receive comprehensive medical care, a "one-stop shop" for virtually any medical problem or need, inpatient or outpatient.

The founders believed that patients benefit when clinicians work together; they also believed in a team model for running the new organization. Physician leaders worked alongside professional managers in making decisions. Early on, the organization developed a reputation for clinical innovation, which is still part of its DNA. The new medical center drew patients from well beyond Seattle; doctors cultivated relationships with physicians in a five-state region and developed a national reputation in several clinical areas. Because the organization always supported education, research, and clinical care, Kaplan has described it as "a sort of halfway house for doctors who were drawn to teach and do research without the publish-or-perish pressures of traditional academic careers."

Today the hospital has 336 beds and 500 physicians who see patients in 9 locations in and around Seattle. There is a strong commitment to graduate medical education; VM supports 4 physician residency programs and a pharmacy residency program. The Benaroya Research Institute on the downtown campus is making breakthrough discoveries in autoimmune disease research. Beginning in 2008, the Virginia Mason Institute began providing education and training in the VMPS to other organizations and healthcare providers.

NEW CHALLENGES

For nearly 80 years, VM enjoyed growth and fiscal health. The late 1990s, however, was a time of unprecedented economic challenges. The growing strain on resources catalyzed the board to think differently about what it would take to thrive once again.

Robert Mecklenburg, MD, a practicing physician, chief of medicine, and a newly appointed board member in 2000, recalls his first board meeting. "I was jolted out of feeling invulnerable. If I looked at the organization through the lens of being a doctor, I felt things were as they had always been—basically good." But at Mecklenburg's first meeting, the board chair and the community members learned that VM was losing money. The distress among board members and leadership led to a quickly organized retreat that changed the course of VM's history. The board examined not just financial performance but also the broader issue of the quality of care the institution provided. They carefully considered the Institute of Medicine's 2000 report, *To Err Is Human*. In an unflinching inward look, the board identified putting the patient first as a core strategy going forward.

Recognizing the Need to Change the Culture

The board asked itself how well an individualistic, physician-oriented culture served the community. In 1986 the physician-owned partnership had been dissolved and all doctors had become employees of a new nonprofit, Virginia Mason Medical Center. The prior nonprofit hospital board essentially became the new medical center board; community members made up the majority of the board, which also included four internal VM members.

Despite this structural change, the physician culture remained pretty much intact. The doctors had inherited the expectations of protection, autonomy, and entitlement. They were not always aligned with acting to benefit colleagues, the organization, or the greater community. Again, Mecklenburg offers his view as a physician member of that board:

> Before VM could build anything new at all, the doctors needed to have a different relationship to the organization and through the organization to the community. The model of physician leader as alderman or "union boss"—to bring resources to physicians from the community (through patients)—had to change. They needed to accept that there is a duty to flow in the opposite direction, to be accountable to the organization and community. In a sense the community was the "new boss" and VM was the conduit through which its physicians served the community.

An Activist Board

The board played a critical role in catalyzing and supporting a deep transformation in the culture and in the provision of healthcare. The board's orientation toward community forced the leadership to look at a picture much bigger than "how do we put more money on the books?" As those who hold fiduciary responsibility, it would have been natural for board members to focus on righting the financial ship at a time of economic loss. But they viewed the economic situation—as well as quality of care and the board's community obligation—as an opportunity to begin something new. At that time, they didn't know what "something new" would be. They didn't come out of their retreat with a blueprint for action but with ideas about what could be changed.

Was it good timing? Serendipity? In the late 1990s, when transformation was needed, the board included individuals with the professional expertise and courage to address the fundamental issues: Who are we? and What do we need to become to serve this community? The board was central to the fundamental changes the organization subsequently made; its members drove home the need to do something different from what had been done in the past.

The CEO

Another piece of the jigsaw puzzle that fell into place at this time was Gary Kaplan's election to CEO. After his medical training at the University of Michigan, Kaplan went west to Seattle in 1978 and climbed the leadership ranks, from section head to chief of satellites and regional clinics to co-chair of medical center operations. In 2000 he became VM's seventh CEO; his predecessor had been in the role for 20 years.

Elections

VM physicians traditionally elected their CEO. Kaplan's election was notable for two reasons: He was the first primary care doctor to be elected CEO in a specialty-oriented medical group, and he represented the newer generation of doctors. Part and parcel of the physician leader's role had always been to deliver for constituents while protecting them from change. Kaplan ran for election not long after a financial downturn that had caused no small amount of angst among the doctors; Hillary Clinton's plans for healthcare reform stirred even more concern. The implications for the VM specialists weren't clear, but it felt to many that change—for the worse—was in the air.

Once elected, Kaplan and a few colleagues raised the issue of a different way to select leaders, which proved to be a pivotal conversation. Board members who were from disciplines other than medicine thought electing leaders was an organizational vulnerability. No other industry with revenues of $700 million would use a political process to select leaders. The board immediately offered to abolish elections and move to appoint the CEO. Kaplan was now in the challenging position of telling colleagues who had just elected him that they would no longer vote for leadership. He asked the board to delay any official policy change for 30 days to give him time to work through the issue with the doctors.

Right away, Kaplan was on the firing line facing outright anger. In one meeting, an irate doctor marched down the aisle and aggressively grabbed the mike to air his resentment. As Kaplan tells it, "Those 30 days were among the most difficult of my 30 years at Virginia Mason. I had doctors I had practiced with come up to me and say, 'You should have said, "Vote for me and I'll take away your vote!"'"

Lead-Up to the September 2000 Retreat

One of Kaplan's campaign promises was to organize a retreat to address doctors' malaise and the economic challenges. It had been five years since the last retreat. In other organizations, the promise of a retreat might not be much of an enticement. But in this particular context—financial challenges, anxiety that the organization had lost its way, and external changes—the opportunity to convene as a group was viewed as significant. Once the board finalized the decision to move away from electing leaders, the retreat's importance grew. The retreat was to be an opportunity to air everyone's issues, look at matters of concern to the board, and turn a page in VM's history. To head the agenda committee, Kaplan chose Joyce Lammert, MD, an allergist who had no formal leadership role but in whom Kaplan saw a future leader. His instinct for talent served the retreat committee and, ultimately, the compact work well.

GENESIS OF A NEW COMPACT

The Idea of Compact

The compact first came into the picture in the course of planning the retreat. Three committee members who had attended Jack Silversin's workshop at the December 1999 Institute for Healthcare Improvement (IHI) annual forum proposed the idea of developing a compact. Donna Smith, MD, whose pediatric group practice had joined VM, recalls, "I just got it. It resonated as a conversation we needed to have at Virginia Mason. The burning platform for us was the need for clarity about the future and the physician's role in the organization." Smith recruited two others for the repeat session of Silversin's workshop: Diane Miller, director of organizational development, and Kim Leatham, MD, a primary care doctor based in the Bainbridge Island satellite clinic. Smith recalls the workshop's main points as being so powerful that she bought the cassette of the talk to share with others. Smith and Leatham suggested the compact as a retreat topic and handed the workshop cassette to Lammert. Smith recalls her approach not as "This is an answer to all of our issues," but rather, "See what you make of this—I think this conversation is important for us to have." The message seemed timely and important.

Lammert wasn't convinced. Initially, she felt that the compact was too "soft" a topic to get the physicians' attention. This retreat was a big deal; it was planned for two days off-site for all physicians. Considerable expense would be involved; given the center's financial performance and everyone's concern for the future, the stakes were high for the new CEO. Only the enthusiasm of those who had been at the IHI workshop led Lammert to speak with Kaplan about incorporating the compact message into the retreat. A phone conference with Silversin was organized before Kaplan and Lammert decided to proceed. Kaplan knew of Silversin's work because both men regularly attended American Medical Group Association conferences and Medical Group Management Association meetings.

Silversin was invited to the retreat with the understanding that the retreat's objective was not to fashion a new compact. The agenda was broader and included clarifying the safety imperative. John Nance, a Seattle-based aviation expert, would tee up that discussion and share the crew resource management approach developed by the airlines to reduce mishaps. The retreat's other objective was to discuss what it means to be a doctor at VM in the twenty-first century.

With that remit, Silversin suggested that he conduct interviews so he could better understand the issues the doctors and the organization were facing. Kaplan recalls, "Initially I did not feel totally comfortable with this. I was still a relatively new chief executive and the idea of some consultant coming in and interviewing doctors and managers was out of the norm. What would he make of what he heard? What would he learn that would be difficult for me to hear? I might not have been entirely comfortable with the plan to conduct interviews, but at that stage I was convinced we had to go forward."

The Retreat

More than 13 years later, doctors with whom I spoke still recall the significance of that retreat. Common recollections are of the communal spirit participants felt and of the venting, loss, and mourning that took place over the two days. Smith remembers, "It was an event. The whole thing worked as a package. Beyond John Nance's content and Jack's discussion, there were skits that people had signed up for in advance. What contributed to a deeper familiarity and vulnerability was that people carpooled to the venue and shared accommodations. It all seemed to build a community feeling." Some recall profound feelings of loss that emerged from the discussion of what VM had been, how it had to change, and what it meant to doctors.

I've noted across many organizations that the opportunity to grieve what's gone is critical to successful compact work. When discussions skim the surface and result largely in lists of what doctors need to do differently and what leaders need to do, something important is missed. The rich meaning that VM's compact has today is the result of the process that developed it. The retreat instigated a deeper examination of the old deal and kicked off a process that involved many meetings, took more than a year, and touched every physician in the organization. This all-important retreat created a safe enough space for doctors to express what they were experiencing.

According to Kaplan, the conversations weren't always easy or comfortable. In an open-discussion period, he and then-president Mike Rona sat on stools in the front of the room while participants lobbed question after question their way. No one held back or tried to be polite. The physicians' candor mattered. The leaders' willingness to hear it mattered. The time away from practice demands and family commitments mattered. To echo Smith's observation, "The whole thing worked as a package."

Discussions

The intention was not to develop a compact during the retreat but to generate discussions and see where those led. Some design elements did help to foster open conversation. Participants worked in small groups, with a peer facilitator at each table. The facilitator was prepped for this role in advance and had a discussion guide as an aid.

The first afternoon, participants discussed what the organization should provide to doctors. The questions to stimulate conversation included the following:

- What communication is lacking today that would make physicians' lives at VM more meaningful and facilitate them to better contribute to the organization?
- What ways, methods, and venues of communicating are most and least meaningful to physicians? Which should be used more? Which should be modified? Which should be eliminated?
- What are the current problems with physician participation? What issues do physicians want to be able to shape or influence? How do they want to participate?

First the tables, then the group at large, debriefed to generate a list of what physicians wanted and needed from the organization.

The next morning, tables discussed what physicians owed VM. Prepared questions generated intense conversation—about the past and what VM had been, and why past success could no longer be counted on to carry the day. These questions included the following:

- What does it mean to be a good citizen of the VM medical group? What are physicians' responsibilities to the organization as a whole?
- What are the standards we should hold VM physicians to regarding their relationships with patients and patients' families?
- How should physicians interact with and lead support staff? What responsibilities do physicians have for setting an example for other staff to follow?
- How should VM physicians relate to other VM physicians? What do we expect from each other? Consider relationships within and across departments.

Perhaps because the conversations were not set up to directly identify "gives" and "gets" in a new compact, they produced a good deal of candor and allowed for heartfelt emotions to be expressed. Not rushing over this step in the process—considering the past and letting go of what isn't helpful to the future—turned out to play a significant part in the acceptance of the compact document that evolved over the coming months.

In verbally evaluating the retreat before it ended, most attendees said that the two days had been worthwhile. However, a few commented that, after similar events, initial enthusiasm had faded and commitments had a tendency to drop off the radar screen. The general consensus was that follow-up should be taken seriously. Using the work accomplished in the retreat to formalize a new compact was seen as desirable and important to most participants.

The Compact

After the retreat, Lammert and Kaplan decided to form a committee charged with developing a new compact. Lammert was again asked to take the lead. Kaplan agreed to be a member to stay in touch with what the organization would commit to do; he was reluctant, however, to be too strong a voice, concerned that expressing his views would sway others or diminish the vigor of debate. Other members included Tom Biehl, MD; Shelly Fagerlund from human resources; Dan Hanson, MD; Dawna Kramer, MD; Kim Leatham, MD; Drew Schembre, MD; Pat Scott, a board member and VM patient; and Joel Wakefield, the medical center attorney.

The Compact Committee
The compact was developed by insiders; Silversin and I played a relatively minor role. We drafted a series of e-mail messages that Kaplan modified and sent to every professional staff member. These messages reminded the retreat attendees about

what was accomplished at the retreat and explained to those who didn't attend what had gone on at the retreat, the basics of a compact, and how VM was going to develop an explicit new deal. Silversin also provided support via telephone to Kaplan and Lammert throughout the process.

The compact committee met at 7 a.m. every other week for nearly a year. This regular contact solidified the group, allowing its members to develop the comfort and safety needed to share candid observations and challenge one another's views.

The first draft of the compact was based on comments captured during the retreat. What emerged was a short list of headings on each "side," with examples of specific behaviors under each. The committee chose not to use give-and-get language, opting instead for the construct of "Organization's Responsibilities" and "Physician's Responsibilities."

For surgeon Tom Biehl, the attraction of the compact was its reciprocal nature. It was not a statement of "here are the rules." In his view, this two-way nature was critical to its acceptance. The fact that the organization's obligations to doctors were stated up front helped secure support for this new deal. Biehl said, "Even the visuals of the document are important. We started by enumerating the organization's responsibilities on the left. Before listing what's expected from doctors, it's better to create some sense of what's in it for them."

From the start, wording was carefully chosen. The committee didn't want the language to be inflammatory or raise hackles. According to Biehl, "As doctors read the headings on their side of the compact, a common response is 'of course.' Those words connect to a doctor's sense of his or her professionalism. While the headings aren't in themselves particularly controversial, the expected behaviors under each are different from the past."

Presenting the Compact

The committee continued to meet until mid-2001 before it felt it had a draft that could be shared widely. Two committee members attended section and department meetings to present the draft and collect reactions and comments. For many on the committee, it was their first experience facing the full range of reactions from colleagues. One skeptical pathologist asked, "Why do we need this? Won't it be used to fire us?" These meetings included not just physicians but physician leaders and managers as well—those closest to the front line, who would be delivering on the organization's commitments.

Group meetings were held throughout the summer, and committee members continued to rework the document based on what they heard. They held a series of presentations and discussions at the management committee (physician and professional administrator executives, chaired by Kaplan) to ensure the organization's responsibilities were acceptable and to give these individuals the opportunity to offer other general input.

The final draft was presented at an all-professional-staff meeting. Based on their experience of both hostile and supportive responses, committee members performed several skits demonstrating specific behaviors the compact was intended to address. Knowing humor would help defuse anger or suspicion, they acted out situations that would resonate with doctors and make them think, "Yes, we need this compact."

After the staff meeting, the management committee officially approved the compact. Exhibit 3.1 shows the categories included in the compact. The full compact is reproduced in the appendix.

Mutual Accountability

The final document spells out a new relationship between the organization and the doctors. It makes explicit that a relationship exists and that each party has duties to the other. It does not comprise a long list of expectations, but for those at VM in 2000–2001, each heading had import and relevance. The examples under each heading are illustrative, not comprehensive. By being both clear and reciprocal, the compact lays the groundwork for mutual accountability. Doctors could now tell leaders, "You're not keeping to your end of this deal." And leaders now felt they had firmer ground to stand on in performance-management conversations with doctors.

Recalling the development of the compact, Lammert says, "It wasn't a thunderclap—it all proceeded in an iterative way. The months put into those discussions and debates made the compact a document with relevance, meaning, and usefulness in moving the organization toward its aims."

Exhibit 3.1 Categories of Responsibilities in the Virginia Mason Medical Center Physician Compact

Organization's Responsibilities	Physician's Responsibilities
Foster Excellence	Focus on Patients
Listen and Communicate	Collaborate on Care Delivery
Educate	Listen and Communicate
Reward	Take Ownership
Lead	Change

Source: Virginia Mason Medical Center. Used with permission.

MOVING FORWARD

Vision

Compact development proceeded nearly in parallel with work to create a vision for the organization's future.

The board encouraged the executive team to put patients front and center in the organization's vision. Board members who were VM patients pointed out that doctors might have *thought* they were putting patients first, but in fact they were organizing care around their own needs, preferences, or traditions. If a doctor didn't get around to discharging a patient on a Friday, why did the patient have to wait until Monday to go home? Why did patients show up at their appointed time only to be told to take a seat until the doctor was ready to see them? Challenges such as these helped Kaplan and his executive team understand how radical it would be if the organization did, in fact, put patients first and built care processes around them. It would upend much of the thinking and practices already being questioned by the compact work.

Strategic Plan

As the distillation of what management, doctors, and staff believe and act on, VM's strategic plan guides all decisions; it is the organization's soul (Exhibit 3.2). Its value is a function of its visibility to one and all. In the decade since it was developed, it has been used continually to choose direction and set priorities. The most common frame for any decision is, "Is this good for patients?" Using the plan in this way sets it apart from the usual mission and vision statements posted on the walls of most care-delivery organizations. The content of the VM strategic plan sounds good *and* serves as a practical guide. Many others just sound good.

Production System

Together, the physician compact and the strategic plan laid the groundwork for the VMPS. Only after the compact was finalized and the strategic plan was developed and communicated did leaders actively seek a methodology to realize their vision of being the leader in healthcare quality.

In June 2002, board members, executives, managers, and doctor leaders made their first site visit to Japan to see the Toyota Production System in action and

Exhibit 3.2 Virginia Mason Strategic Plan

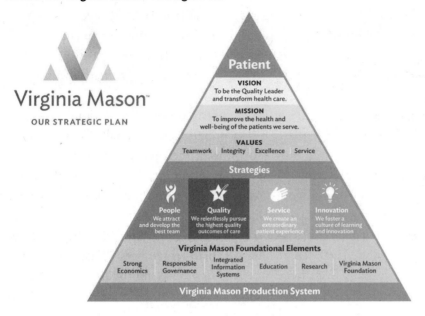

study how it could be applied to their medical center. After that trip, executives committed to what would become their management system: VMPS. They became students of Chihiro Nakao (one of only two living disciples of Taiichi Ohno), who today still serves as their *sensei* (teacher). After two weeks in Japan, Kaplan and the others on that initial journey were "all in."

Meaningful Change Is Difficult

John Kotter and Dan Cohen (2002) coined the phrase "see, feel, change" to represent the process by which most people adopt change. The critical word is "feel"—not "think about" or "read a report." Emotional experiences propel change. This fact accounts for the impact of the Japan trip on those who participated. Andrew Jacobs, MD, VM's current medical director for physician engagement and leadership development, had a critical insight on the initial trip about the connection between Lean and his practice of medicine:

> At the Hitachi plant producing air conditioners, I was assigned to observe and study all the movements of one operator whom I'll always remember as "Operator No. 3." In the process of focusing on this one individual, I had an epiphany. . . . I saw myself as Operator No. 3. I instantly translated the chain of events that produced

an air conditioner unit into the process of which I, as an oncologist, am a part. I could see that I work downstream from others and that what I'm able to do for any one patient is affected by those upstream. The outcomes for any patient I treat would only be as good as the weakest link in the chain. This is true in any production process, clinical ones included.

Pushback from those who did not make the trip was fast and furious. From the start, some staff members saw the trip as a boondoggle. A small group, angered by what they viewed as a waste of resources, took their story to the local press as the group was starting the trip. When Kaplan announced the organization was committed to adopting the Toyota Production System, the expected reactions were voiced: "Patients are not cars," "This might apply to primary care but has no place in surgery," "You're talking about cookie-cutter medicine," "No way does this make sense for us in the legal department." Kaplan remembers, "Responses to the message we brought back from Japan were distributed along the bell curve. About 10 percent had genuine enthusiasm. Another 10 percent declared, 'Over my dead body,' while the majority of staff and doctors were in the middle, many ambivalent but most adopting a wait-and-see attitude."

One Example of Kaizen

There are countless examples of how VM has eliminated waste from processes, saved money, and improved patient care. Biehl gives one example: standardizing surgical instrument setups. For a complex operation, central supply would sterilize, and technicians would organize, two hundred to three hundred instruments on a tray when, on average, only 10 percent of them are used. This exercise represented a waste of materials and waste of employees' time and effort. Through a *kaizen* event, the number of instruments was reduced to the critical few. This change required the cooperation of doctors; for instance, to standardize the tray for gallbladder removal, all surgeons had to agree on what was needed. Biehl believes the vision and compact made a significant difference in doctors' willingness to get involved and get on board when others work out new systems.

Strong Leadership

How did such a radical message take hold and result in the success of the VMPS evident today?

My view, confirmed by those I spoke with, is that both the strategic plan and the physician compact paved the way. But the *most important* factor was leaders' courage to reference the compact and strategic plan and their determination to help others better understand the organization's direction and to participate in change.

Kaplan's position was that not everyone had to be a champion for change, but nobody could be an obstacle. Kaplan also had a growing understanding that there were going to be losses:

> At first it was very difficult for me to accept that colleagues I had respect for and had practiced with would put up roadblocks to what I saw as essential to this organization's success. Once I appreciated that this wasn't for everyone, it was easier to truly honor the service they had provided and make it easy for them to find work elsewhere. Of course, some didn't go quietly or easily. In the end 5 to 10 percent, some for totally unrelated reasons, left in the early years of the journey.

Focusing on the Compact

Lammert took the lead in ensuring that the compact did not fade from view. Each month for the first two years, she e-mailed all providers a short written piece called "Compact College" that highlighted a different compact element. Most tips were aimed at making physicians' practice easier (e.g., phone shortcuts). For the most part, she focused on what the organization had committed to, but at times also wrote about physicians' responsibilities. A popular resource Lammert provided was a pre-vacation to-do list summarizing steps providers needed to take to inform others that they would be out of the office.

In 2009, Andrew Jacobs, VM's then–chief medical officer (CMO), began the practice of ending each monthly professional staff meeting with an unstructured discussion of a tenet from the compact. This meeting starts at the end of the practice day and runs for an hour and a half; typically, between 50 and 90 people attend. Jacobs chose to start by exploring views on the organization's commitments. In many compact processes we've been a part of, doctors feel that holding them accountable is easy, but they question what opportunities they have to hold leadership to account.

Jacobs found a thirst for these conversations. He sees them as a means not just to keep the compact in front of the professional staff but also to engage them in it. Because, from the start, his meetings focused on how well the organization was holding up its end of the deal, he sent a signal that leadership takes its own commitments as seriously as it holds doctors to theirs. Jacobs offers an example: "'Create opportunities to participate in or support research' is in our compact, but when that was the discussion topic, people opened up that they felt we were not doing enough in this area. This and other candid discussions proved to be powerful indicators that the organization was willing to openly hear views and support civil dialogue."

Today, professional staff meetings still end with open discussions that aren't held in any other venue and are now "standard work"—an expected part of the agenda. These regular discussions are one way to reinforce that leaders are expected to live by their compact responsibilities; the meetings allow doctors a chance to express concerns and leaders to get direct, honest feedback. Discussions have broadened to include philosophical or ethical questions relative to the practice of medicine. Jacobs feels that this opportunity continues to tap into something deep that VM physicians need.

HARDWIRING THE COMPACT

To optimize the value of a compact process, VM, like most organizations, turned to human resources processes to hardwire or stabilize the changes into organizational life.

Hiring People Committed to the Organization's Vision and Mission

The acceptance and use of the compact wasn't a straight-upward trend line. VM went through a period of increased physician turnover in the first few years after the compact and strategic plan were adopted. Jacobs concluded that the organization did not pay enough attention to recruits' cultural fit, that he and other leaders focused too much on accomplishments listed on curricula vitae. After their realization, department chiefs and section heads increased their efforts to find people who supported the organization's direction.

It's natural that during the early stages there were more mismatches in hiring than there are today. The joining-up process for new doctors—which leaders tried to make as clear as possible—might not have sufficiently spelled out all the ways VM was different from other organizations. Some doctors had left VM, some would eventually leave, and some skeptics became advocates for the changes. The new patient-centric culture was still gelling; who "fit" into it was not yet clear. And culture change is a long process.

More than 13 years on, the contrast between VM and other healthcare providers is clear—and the gap wide. The now-obvious distinctions make it easier to select those who will support the culture, the compact, and the VMPS.

Physician and Leadership Recruitment
Doctors who express interest in a position at VM receive a letter from Kaplan that thanks them for their interest and includes the physician compact. Being clear at

the very start helps VM focus its recruitment efforts on those who choose to work there after having read the compact. Leaders are also selected for their willingness and capability to fulfill the organization's side of the compact and the commitments detailed in the leadership compact (discussed later in this chapter).

Physician Orientation

CMO Michael Glenn describes the compact's utility in physician orientation as follows:

> The compact is a valuable tool for communicating, up front, what the expectations are both ways. It provides solid footing for the relationship doctors can expect to have here at VM. In the first conversations with a new hire, he or she is taking in a lot of information and there's usually not any pushback, questions, or even discussion about it. It's presented—and taken—as a routine part of getting on board. *And* this is not the first time a doctor is hearing about it. Any recruit who comes through sees it, and it is gone over in the recruitment process. Onboarding represents a second "touch."

Glenn sums up the essence of the deal: By giving up complete autonomy, you get a system that supports your practice, is predictable, and helps make you efficient. You give up something, but you get something important and valuable in return. The clarity of the exchange captured in the compact is different from anything in this organization's past.

Reviewing the compact during orientation isn't limited to the doctors that VM employs. Other physicians who have admitting privileges at VM also are shown the compact in their VM orientation, and their accountability is explained. While about 50 VM doctors were oriented in 2010, more than double (approximately 120) from other organizations were oriented to the compact. Glenn states, "For those doctors we don't employ, the compact is equally or more relevant. It's a critical tool for letting doctors know what is expected of them while they are caring for patients here."

Compact in Action

In Mecklenburg's words, the compact work "normalized and narrowed acceptable behavior. Its strength is that it was written by doctors. . . . It sets out 'this is how we act.'"

In a relatively short time, the "old boys' club" culture began to shift. One female doctor recalls VM's sixtieth anniversary celebration at which one physician stand-up comic remarked, "The Center for Women's Health has been so successful that leadership is thinking we should start a Center for Men's Health . . . until they realized that's what it had always been!" No one could imagine such disrespectful remarks being made publicly today. Having more female doctors and primary care doctors has added diversity, while using the compact as the basis for feedback has helped shift norms.

Physician leaders point to the compact as an essential part of performance discussions. CMO Glenn says, "The compact gives me a way to talk about things when giving feedback to doctors. It depersonalizes feedback and takes away any hint of 'I'm judging you.' This is about agreements being made. Not 'I'm coming down on you.'"

As chief of primary care, Catherine Potts is responsible for all primary care providers across nine sites. Rarely has she had to pull out her copy of the compact and point out a specific part to a physician. But she does bring it to every performance review and, as the meeting concludes, Potts hands it to the doctor and thanks him or her for contributions in the past year. Potts also references the utility of having the compact as the organization moves toward population management, a move that brings stresses for primary care doctors. While most patients don't need to see a physician for an upper respiratory tract infection—they can be managed by other practitioners or over the phone—doctors are reluctant to give up the "easy" appointments. According to Potts, conversations about new care models are opportunities to remind doctors that participating in organizational change is part of the deal.

Tom Biehl, the section head of general thoracic and vascular surgery, makes regular use of the printed document. "When I can point to the organization's compact commitments, it's easier to get doctor agreement to do something. 'I'm asking you to do this *and* this is what you get out of this'." Among the physician leaders I spoke with, "showing respect for all" was cited as the most common compact violation. Biehl commented, "It's enough to call it out when breaches happen. I don't have to pull out a hard copy of the compact and point out how a behavior is 'off-compact' for every minor infraction; by now doctors know that disrespectful behavior isn't going to be tolerated."

COMPENSATION

As chair of VM's compensation committee for several years, Joyce Lammert was in a key position to carry on the compact work she had begun as chair of the original compact committee. Her commitment—along with others'—to sustain the compact has led to experimenting with increasing the compensation earned for citizenship.

The compensation formula includes a portion for what VM calls PAGE—professional activities and group effort.[1] Since compact implementation, "group effort" has been more clearly defined; its categories are based on the compact. Staff give input via 360-degree feedback surveys on all providers; the section head factors that input into each provider's group-effort assessment. Those with scores above the medical center mean for group effort and professional activity are financially rewarded.

VM's primary care compensation is moving away from its emphasis on productivity to a closer alignment with quality-score metrics. The goal is to increase the percentage of compensation based on quality scores and citizenship, largely defined by participation in organizational change.

NEW ROLES FOR ALL PHYSICIANS

Physician Leaders

After 2000, all physician leaders were appointed. At that time, 18 section heads reported to Chief of Medicine Mecklenburg, who let them know that their job description had changed. His message was: Our job is now change management and bringing section members to accept a new approach to healthcare delivery. According to Mecklenburg, "This was a substantive change in job description for me as well as for each section head. I was careful to convey that I would be making the same choice and transition as an individual as they would be making." He also told them, "We will learn how to do this together. You can choose to not step into this different role. If this is unappealing, we still honor you and you'll be able to continue in your clinical and academic roles." Sixteen section heads opted out or were replaced within three years. According to Mecklenburg, this was rarely traumatic. It was simply a matter of identifying where each individual could be most effective while choosing the clinical leaders necessary for the organization's new direction.

Physicians

As a speaker for events sponsored by TransforMed—a subsidiary of the American Academy of Family Practice that helps practices to become patient-centered medical homes—Kim Leatham, MD, shares the work she led to implement VM's "medical home," or primary care model.

In her talks, Leatham emphasizes that the changes needed for a medical home to work require a new compact or some other way to create culture change. A common response from her audience is, "We couldn't do that—we'd lose half our doctors." The fear of losing doctors, Leatham feels, is a bullet leaders have to bite, and having a compact makes it easier to make difficult decisions. A compact paves the way for doctors either to create and accept new ways of working, or to leave when it's clear they won't get on board with the change.

Formerly the leader at her practice site, Leatham reflects on a significant leadership lesson: "You can't exist in a paradigm in which the leader's job is to make doctors happy. Because that isn't how I saw my job, the unhappy ones have gone—by choice or not. Now I have my ideal practice, and I have satisfied colleagues. The irony is the happiness that all of us now experience has resulted from our collective stepping away from the old compact."

IMPACT OF THE PHYSICIAN COMPACT ON NURSES

I asked Charleen Tachibana, chief nursing officer at VM, if having a compact with physicians affected nursing staff. She replied:

> The physician compact is one of the best things that happened to nurses in the organization. We had a need to change our culture, which in the past was physician focused. They set the culture because they had power in the organization—their actions mattered in shaping the culture and keeping it going. And the other group that shaped culture was leadership. We have both a physician and leadership compact because those two groups are the key ones in setting the tone for all others. It's not that others don't matter, but these two groups have the most impact, and the compacts [leadership and physician] have leveraged the influence of these two to reshape our culture.

Tachibana feels that the physician compact and leadership compact (described on pages 39–41) are of equal importance in moving the organization toward its goals. "Our compacts haven't aged," she said. "They captured values felt at the time to be important to a new culture and these have endured."

AFTER ALL THESE YEARS

In his role as medical director for physician engagement and leadership development, Jacobs has wondered if it's time to refresh the physician compact. When we spoke, he noted that 13 years had gone by and the organization had undergone a visible transformation since the physician compact was developed. Still, about the compact, Jacobs concludes, "Nothing has outlived its usefulness and nothing is missing."

With the compact's focus on patient-centeredness, respect, innovation, and continuous learning, he described the compact as "eerily prescient" of the production-system work that followed its adoption. In part, the continued relevance of the compact is a result of the time and attention devoted to crafting something that addressed immediate concerns and that would be resilient for years to come. It's interesting to consider, much as Jacobs noted, that the compact so accurately foreshadowed the environment the VMPS would need to thrive. Perhaps serendipity also played a small part.

THE VIRGINIA MASON LEADERSHIP COMPACT

VM's unique leadership compact was developed after the physician compact and as an outgrowth of the strategic plan.

The first iteration of the strategic plan had four pillars, still unchanged: people, quality, service, and innovation. In 2001, each pillar had a point person who led teams to expand that pillar's initial content and define a five-year proposal for it. Diane Miller was the director of organizational development; she was concentrating on leadership development when the people pillar of the strategic plan was being built.

As she recalls, a group consisting of executives, physician leaders, and managers—including key leaders of the physician compact—were asked to address "leadership" as one part of the people-pillar strategies. "We wondered if the headings in the doctor compact could form the basis of a leadership compact," she said. This group explored the idea and generated headings and possible content to produce the first draft of the leadership compact. The next draft developed from a series of town hall meetings for all leaders. It took about nine months to finalize the leadership compact. At that point, the group that had created and vetted the leadership compact took it to CEO Kaplan and the then-president to review and "bless" it.

Miller says, "The leadership compact is now a part of 'who we are.' The principles in it are in sync with production-system work, and it has real meaning" (Exhibit 3.3). The leadership compact is shown at the monthly managers' meeting led by Sarah Patterson, the executive vice president and chief operating officer, who calls out the organizational responsibility to which the topic under discussion relates. As with the physician compact, the leadership version is used to recruit managers and leaders and serves as the basis of performance reviews.

In the years since its original development, the parties have made one change to the compact. "Be a problem solver" was originally on the "leader" side of the compact. New language acknowledges that frontline doctors and staff also are expected to solve problems. The work of leaders has shifted: They are now expected to be facilitators and coaches, and not the ones to swoop in and solve the problems.

Exhibit 3.3 Excerpt from Virginia Mason Medical Center Leadership Compact

Organization Responsibilities	Leader Responsibilities
Foster Excellence ◆ Recruit and retain the best people ◆ Acknowledge and reward contributions to patient care and the organization ◆ Provide opportunities for growth of leaders ◆ Continuously strive to be the quality leader in health care ◆ Create an environment of innovation and learning **Lead and Align** ◆ Create alignment with clear and focused goals and strategies ◆ Continuously measure and improve our patient care, service, and efficiency ◆ Manage and lead organization with integrity and accountability ◆ Resolve conflict with openness and empathy ◆ Ensure safe and healthy environment and systems for patients and staff	**Focus on Patients** ◆ Promote a culture where the patient comes first in everything we do ◆ Continuously improve quality, safety, and compliance **Promote Team Medicine** ◆ Develop exceptional working-together relationships that achieve results ◆ Demonstrate the highest levels of ethical and professional conduct ◆ Promote trust and accountability within the team

Source: Virginia Mason Medical Center. Used with permission.

Cathie Furman, senior vice president for quality and compliance, spoke with me about the usefulness of the leadership compact in selecting managers and executives who "fit" with the VM culture. Furman feels that the match issue is as critical for leaders in the organization as it is for physicians. The higher a leader is in the hierarchy, the higher the cost is to recruit and replace that individual. Of course, the many people who report to that individual are greatly affected by his or her values, decisions, and actions. Moving someone out of a position is hugely disruptive. "The leadership compact is as central to moving the organization forward on its strategic plan as the physician compact is," emphasizes Furman.

In my experience, VM's leadership compact is unique. For the reasons discussed, it clearly has added value to the healthcare organization. This kind of compact would be particularly helpful in organizations that are transitioning to including more advanced physician leaders. Chiefs and department heads are better able to step up and lead when they know the organization has their backs. Making a clear deal with current and emerging leaders is useful in addressing the difficulties they face when colleagues accuse them of "crossing over" to management's camp. In essence, a new deal for leaders is one that says: We know that leadership is risky business; in exchange for your stepping up and taking a leadership role, we will help you develop skills and will support you in multiple ways.

Virginia Mason Medical Center: *Kaizen* in the Boardroom

At Virginia Mason Medical Center (VM), *kaizen* is applied not only to processes in the hospital, clinic, and support services, but also to processes in the boardroom. The board constantly strives to improve how it governs. While the medical center pursues its quest for the perfect patient experience, the board has engaged in a parallel process to become increasingly sophisticated in its ability to support this bold vision. Adopting a written organization–board compact has played a significant role.

Carolyn Corvi, chair of the board from 2009 to 2012, was a board member from the early days of VM's adoption of its production system. According to Corvi, "Having this compact reinforces the ongoing nature of governance. It's not just an activity that takes place when we're meeting—each of us has responsibilities when we're in the community. Every member has to be an advocate for VM outside of meetings. That gives us as board members more to think about. It has really redefined what governance entails."

Virginia Mason's Transformation Leads to Board Compact

In 2000, expectations of board members were still implicit. CEO Gary Kaplan, MD, describes this unarticulated compact this way: "As was typical, our board members saw their primary role as hiring or firing the CEO, attending meetings, and helping define strategy. In those days, quality wasn't necessarily the purview of the board—that was left to the medical staff. If board members held onto that traditional view, they could not be as helpful as we needed given the transformation we had begun."

Board members wanted the institution to provide high-quality, safe care; either they themselves were patients or their family members were. They got satisfaction out of serving, and the organization benefitted from their expertise when finances trended downward in the late 1990s. The decisions executive leadership made to put forward a bold vision and adopt the Virginia Mason Production System represented a departure from business as usual; everyone from the board to frontline staff had a part to play in the transformation.

Understanding the Need for Change

Several board members participated in the initial two-week study tour of Japanese factories that Kaplan had organized to better understand Lean processes and their applicability to healthcare. Corvi felt the Japan trips were unique experiences. She remarked, "It's intense and hard work. The group [leaders, board members, doctors, staff] is together for two weeks, nearly 24 hours a day. You get to know people in a very different way. Those experiences help us be more effective board members." Board members benefit not just from the bonding and insights into the work others do, but also from firsthand experience with the Lean tools that colleagues at the medical center would need to master. Today, going on the annual Japan study tour during their first term is a prerequisite for board member term renewal.

New Roles

The bar for board membership has been raised since that first trip. In Kaplan's words:

> For our board to lead us to achieve the vision they had helped develop—to put patients first and provide the best care, anywhere—those on the board would need to see their role differently and partner with the executive team differently. Accountability was increasingly important as we began to make Virginia Mason Production System our management system. Accountability had to be modeled at the board level, and the board needed to hold me and my team to standards higher than ever before.

The Board Compact

The development and adoption of the organization–board compact was an offshoot of the physician and leadership compacts. Those compacts provided board members with models for how explicit, reciprocal expectations can be assets as their own work evolved and new members joined. Developed over a few meetings by the board, the organization–board compact specifies both board members' and the organization's obligations. The compact is reproduced in its entirety in the appendix. Exhibit 3.4 highlights the headings under the organization's and the board member's responsibilities:

Exhibit 3.4 Headings from Virginia Mason Medical Center Board Compact

Organization's Responsibilities	Board Member's Responsibilities
Foster Excellence	Know the Organization
Listen and Communicate	Focus on the Future
Educate	Listen and Communicate
Lead	Take Ownership
	Promote Effective Change

Source: Virginia Mason Medical Center. Used with permission.

Using the Compact

The compact is fundamental to the board's work. Its importance is signaled by its inclusion in every board packet since adoption of the VM strategic plan. Corvi found it valuable to start each meeting by asking someone to read a few lines from the compact and to talk about their meaning. She makes the following point:

> Doing this sets the tone for behavior in the meeting. It might seem obvious, but speaking aloud some part of the compact is different. It means a lot more when we speak it and talk about it. At Boeing, where I worked in executive positions for 34 years, the CEO of Boeing Commercial Airplanes began our weekly meetings by reviewing a point from our "Working Together Principles and Practices." Each executive did this in turn at our own staff meetings. So it seemed entirely natural for me to use the board compact in much the same way.

Joining the board demands a real commitment. Every potential board candidate gets a copy of the compact, and the nominating committee takes the lead in discussing it to ensure a good fit between current members and candidates. The compact helps the board attract and select individuals who want to be active participants and share their expertise or knowledge.

For most organizations, it is not the usual practice to evaluate uncompensated, voluntary board members. But this board has a different mind-set; evaluation of governance and of individual members is taken seriously and based on the compact. At the close of each board meeting, there is a discussion of how well the board lived up to its commitments—but also how management did relative to its own responsibilities. In addition, VM conducts annual full-board self-evaluations, end-of-term chair and member performance evaluations, and evaluation of the chair-elect before he or she moves into the role of chair.

Perhaps most important, the board compact emphasizes good governance on the part of every member, not just the governance subcommittee. The compact makes clear that the success of every meeting is a shared responsibility.

Broad Perspective and Skills: Assets of Hiring from Outside

Only an educated and demanding board is considered helpful. The compact spells out as a board responsibility "To foster innovation and continuous improvement." One innovation is recruiting board members from outside the local community.

Traditionally, community boards govern on behalf of, and are composed of, community members. But, increasingly, the skills needed to govern in the healthcare realm might not reside in the community. It can also be harder for community members to make tough calls that might be necessary for longer term success (closing a service, taking action against a popular doctor). Outsiders whose only focus is the institution's best interests can be an asset.

At this time, VM's board has two members who neither work nor live in Washington state. Jamie Orlikoff, a nationally recognized expert on healthcare governance, joined in 2006. The board shared the compact with him when he was recruited, and he recalls, "It made a big impression on me as I had not ever seen a board one before; I was only previously familiar with physician compacts. I immediately liked the notion of shared responsibility and shared accountability." Corvi describes Orlikoff's appointment as "bringing a depth and breadth of experience that helped further mature the board. He asked us provocative questions like, 'Are we where we want to be?'"

A Living Document of Real Value

"The compact," according to Orlikoff, "performs a service in setting boundaries that produce creative tension. Sometimes our actions as a board bump up against these fixed expectations. Then we ask if the behavior is really out of bounds or if circumstances have changed, calling for a revision in some aspect of the compact or in a procedure."

Earlier under this compact, it was management's responsibility to provide orientation for board members. The governance committee questioned whether management was as well situated as board members to orient new members. Now, board members do the orientation. As a living document, the compact can and has changed as just described. The compact also has brought change to the board, including who's on the board, the degree of accountability that members all feel, and the board's sophistication in carrying out its responsibilities.

According to Corvi, "Having our compact contributes significantly to our governance effectiveness. In other organizations, the executives and board members would have to be willing to sit down and do the work to sort out what each party's obligations should be. That in itself can be challenging work, but the return on investment is there—if everyone then uses it." Orlikoff, who has worked with boards across the country, hasn't yet seen another example of a board's adopting this tool. He has recommended it, but he reports, "Mostly I get quizzical looks. It could be of great value but a board would need to know and deeply understand the compact. That's more likely if the organization has done the work to create a meaningful physician compact. And the board would need to be on its own journey to get more sophisticated."

The commitment to continual improvement—to *kaizen*—has to be there. A compact that defines reciprocal expectations between board members and the organization is a tool to support the felt need and the will to get better and to keep getting better.

SUMMING UP

Some physicians at VM referred to the compact work as a "cultural revolution." In leaders' minds, that work paved the way for the transformative embrace of production system tools and methodology. VM's experience holds lessons both for leaders aspiring to guide game-changing innovation and for those who need to set the stage for more incremental change.

One takeaway from VM's compact work is the requirement for courage, consistency, and taking the long view. Note that the CEO who started the transformation more than a decade ago is still at the helm. Kaplan, the board, and other key leaders appreciated that the transformation they were looking for would be a decade-long project. Holding that perspective is extremely useful. Other success factors include the following:

- VM leaders organized a retreat, attended by well over half the doctors, at which they introduced the compact concept. Key to its success was their creating enough psychological safety so that participants could, and did, communicate frustration and loss over what was changing in their organization.
- VM had total and visible leadership endorsement of the compact development effort. The CEO made it clear he was 100 percent behind the work; he served on the committee that guided the process, yet he allowed others to take the lead—while never backing away from his role as sponsor.
- A committee of doctors, managers, and a patient (who was also a board member) owned the key work of vetting the compact within the organization. The active involvement of a board member helped keep all conversations honest and did not let physicians think a behavior was patient-centered when the average patient would not see it that way.
- Leaders devoted sufficient time—more than a year—to the development and vetting of the compact, which helped physicians let go of some old expectations. The process wasn't rushed to meet a deadline. Multiple conversations, over time, helped mind-sets shift. Still, that much time and conversation didn't reset everyone's expectations. The process did help to "unfreeze" old expectations, but only time and experience embedded new ones.
- In communicating about the compact, focus was placed on first laying out the organization's responsibilities to physicians. VM began the practice of concluding professional staff meetings with an open discussion of how well the leaders were keeping those commitments. This practice helps ease concern that the effort is all about putting physicians under the microscope.

- Once the compact was finalized, communication did not end. Leaders made efforts to keep it in front of doctors and managers. Written communication with reminders and aids were sent. The compact became hardwired into human resources processes.
- The compact was not used in isolation to support the production system work and other change initiatives. It and the strategic plan are viewed as synergistic. The strategic plan in this organization became the raison d'être for continued focus on the compact.
- Last, accountability for living up to compact responsibilities is taken seriously. The compact is the basis of performance feedback. Leaders demonstrated courage by helping doctors who could not embrace the compact to leave VM.

NOTE

1. VM began using PAGE 40 years ago; how "professional activities and group effort" are evaluated and valued has evolved in the years since. Previously, PAGE had been tracked, but criteria for salary adjustments were not totally transparent. "Professional activities" used to include giving talks, doing research, and being involved with committees. "Group effort" was originally defined as citizenship.

CHAPTER 4

ThedaCare Physicians: Integrating Existing Practices into a Healthcare System

HEALTHCARE REFORM STIMULATES PHYSICIAN EMPLOYMENT

Does the following sound familiar? Could it describe a challenge your organization has faced?

Healthcare reform is on everyone's mind: physicians, insurers, hospital executives, government officials, even consumers. The effort to expand insurance coverage to more Americans has become a political football. Televised messages directed to the public confuse, obfuscate, and even scare. This pending reform, along with underlying market changes, provokes hospitals to seriously consider "buy or make" strategies with regard to must-have services.

Against a good deal of uncertainty, hospital leadership buys local practices assuming that strong affiliations with doctors will be essential to stability. Buying practices is seen as a better option than letting them migrate to a competing system.

Independent-minded doctors are brought into the fold as employees. Buyout terms vary slightly depending on factors such as practice desirability, location, and past history with the hospital. The deals offered during the courting process signal that "not very much will really change." The tacit message is, "Your independence will be honored." Even if that's not exactly what hospital leadership means or says, that's what's heard. Or perhaps that is essentially the promise—since system expansion is unprecedented and the players on this field might not appreciate how independence can thwart the achievement of the system's performance goals.

For some time after the buyouts, the autonomy the practices enjoy isn't a barrier to system performance. But with a greater push to raise performance and with a branding strategy that makes consistency across the system more necessary, practice autonomy becomes a liability. System-level leaders challenge the practices to come together and perform as a team. Alignment and tight coordination—essential if the system is to succeed—don't appear on the surface to be difficult to achieve; but experience proves them to be elusive.

When the call for greater systemness comes, it doesn't happen in an emotionally neutral arena. Because of murky expectations and some ill-timed and inadequately thought-through human resources policy changes, the physicians have a jaundiced view of the system's motives. Trust is ruptured. No one is happy—not the providers; not the practice leaders, who are in an untenable situation as practice "representatives"; and not system leaders, who are frustrated that employed providers aren't lined up behind the organization's initiatives.

While this scenario may have a contemporary ring to it, it describes the situation at ThedaCare Physicians circa 1995.

In the mid-1990s, sensing change was inevitable—with or without legislation—hospitals bought primary care practices. Even though "Harry and Louise" television commercials had helped undo Americans' confidence in President Clinton's Health Security Act of 1993, momentum was still behind the acquisition of physician practices. ThedaCare, which at the time was a two-hospital system based in Neenah and Appleton, Wisconsin, decided to secure a base and employ primary care providers. By purchasing existing practices, ThedaCare created ThedaCare Physicians, its primary care division. For about five years the practices were allowed to carry on more or less as usual. By 2000, though, forming more than a nominal system had become a priority. For reasons explored in the following pages, the trust between the system and its employed providers had eroded; just when the relationship needed to be strong and respectful, it was crumbling.

The dynamics that led a hospital system to acquire independent doctors in eastern Wisconsin in the mid-1990s are playing out today across much of the United States. This story explains how a compact between ThedaCare and its employed physicians put the system's primary care division on a new footing, enhanced trust between physicians and the system, and today helps sustain the remarkable quality performance the system now routinely achieves.

WHEN IS AN INTEGRATED DELIVERY SYSTEM NOT A SYSTEM?

Situated in the Lower Fox River Valley in northeastern Wisconsin are numerous cities along the western side of Lake Winnebago extending to the lake's northern reaches. They compose ThedaCare's predominant service area. The towns of Appleton, Neenah, Menasha, Kimberly, Little Chute, and Kaukauna have been important in the paper industry for almost 150 years. In 1872, the multinational Kimberly-Clark Corporation was founded in Neenah to run paper mills.

One of the two anchor hospitals in the ThedaCare system was built in 1909 to honor Theda Clark Peters, the daughter of Charles B. Clark, cofounder of the company that bears his name; the other anchor hospital, Appleton Medical Center, opened in 1958 as a not-for-profit community hospital. In 1987, the two hospitals merged to form Novus Health Group, which changed its name to ThedaCare in 1999. By then, development of an integrated health system was well under way. Typical of delivery system formation, the ThedaCare hospitals became the core with a "wraparound" network of primary care providers and some specialists. In the early 1990s, ThedaCare partnered with local physicians to develop Touchpoint Health Plan, a health maintenance organization that was sold in 2004 to Minnesota-based UnitedHealthcare.

Today the ThedaCare system encompasses 5 hospitals (3 critical access); 27 clinic locations; behavioral health; home health; and a senior living community that includes assisted living and a nursing facility. There are 108 primary care physicians (family practice, pediatrics, internal medicine), 63 associate providers (nurse practitioners and physician assistants), and 119 employed specialists (including physicians and associate providers). Most of the medical staff members at the hospitals are independent practitioners. In early 2014, ThedaCare declared its intention to affiliate with 2 local systems. When those arrangements are finalized, 2 more critical access hospitals will be incorporated along with additional physician clinics and staff.

Buyouts of Physician Practices

In 1995, ThedaCare was making its first foray into primary care through the purchase of several primary care practices. (The majority were family practice physicians, with a few internists.) Acquiring these practices was a route to tighter care integration and a way to ensure the ongoing stability of existing relationships. A pediatric practice was created, not bought, and the division of primary care, ThedaCare Physician Services, was created. Each practice had its unique culture, and in the process of building the division, some variation occurred among practices with regard to acquisition of assets and goodwill. All practices, however, had the same five-year unwind clause. In 2000, doctors in the first of the acquired practices could leave, and a few did, most of those from one practice.

The Changes Begin: Trust Erodes

In the early days, being part of the system didn't require much change from the doctors. The system's quality, as measured by HEDIS (Healthcare Effectiveness Data and Information Set) scores, had always been good. Gregory Long, MD, division medical director at the time, ties these results to local physicians' part-ownership of Touchpoint Health Plan. According to Long, because they played an active role in managing Touchpoint, local doctors were, on the whole, savvy about quality. In both 2002 and 2003, the plan was named the "nation's top clinical performer" by the National Committee for Quality Assurance.

Improving Access

Early on, ThedaCare's commitment to improvement led to its involvement with the Institute for Healthcare Improvement (IHI) Idealized Design of Clinical Office Practices (IDCOP) collaborative. The practice Long was in served as an alpha site to test the IHI IDCOP open-access concept.

In the first few years of the 2000s, access to primary care providers became an issue that pointed to widening fissures between the system's expectations and those of the practices. Approximately five years after becoming ThedaCare employees, doctors still worked a four-day week and cherished their day off. At the same time, however, Touchpoint was growing and bringing more patients into the system. Local employers expected their workers to have access to doctors, but waiting times for routine care became unacceptable. While two practice sites did have success with the open-access model they piloted for IHI, ThedaCare had not been able to implement and sustain same-day appointments for those wanting them across the system. ThedaCare wanted to be able to meet the patients' needs for access when *they* wanted to be seen. In the absence of a patient-focused culture, innovations such as open access are taken up by those physicians who personally gravitate toward them, while they're viewed by others as "management's agenda."

Electronic Medical Records

After enjoying security and a good deal of independence as part of ThedaCare, physicians began to receive a new message: Working on system aims needs to be a priority. Improving access was one shot across their bow; another was the requirement to implement Epic, the electronic medical record (EMR) software, system wide. Beginning in 1999, ThedaCare helped to build Epic functionality, so some practices were involved as early implementers. With enough kinks worked out, leaders felt that, for maximum benefit, the EMR had to be implemented simultaneously across the system, and they designed a rollout strategy. For the doctors who assumed that their responsibilities were to see patients and provide good care, this new requirement—implemented without their input—was seen as a violation. The cries went up: "This is being done *to* me"; "I don't see the benefit for me"; "I don't know how." Such reactions slowed the spread of the EMR across all clinic sites and indicated doctors' growing frustration with new realities.

Selling Touchpoint

ThedaCare made the decision to sell Touchpoint, a move that left the doctors bereft in ways that had not been anticipated. Nearly a decade after the fact, selling the health plan is vividly described as a turning point in the doctors' relationship with ThedaCare. Without Touchpoint, physicians were removed from decisions about what constituted quality and what would be included in contracts. Their direct involvement in those discussions had given the local medical community some degree of influence in an area that mattered to them. They had felt in charge of, not at the mercy of, a significant insurer in their market. The health plan also served as the glue for the local physicians who owned shares in the enterprise that managed the plan on a day-to-day basis. When the plan they had helped found and make successful was sold, many doctors felt anger and loss.

Hospitalist Program

Instituting a hospitalist program was another game changer for primary care. The program improved the quality of practice life for most primary care doctors, and most of them realized personal advantages. However, as other hospitals' experiences bear out, using hospitalists also disrupts long-standing relationships. When doctors have little need to be in the hospital, collegial conversations are missed; the feeling of being connected to the larger enterprise is diminished. Communication with primary care practices, on the whole, gets more challenging. All this was true for ThedaCare—creating a bit more distance between office-based primary care and others in the system.

BUILDING A SYSTEM: EARLY ATTEMPTS

Lean Practices

In 2002, then-CEO John Toussaint, MD, put ThedaCare on a path that many then saw as radical but that has made this system a perennial top performer in quality and safety measures. He and other senior leaders began a serious investigation of

Lean manufacturing and concluded that ThedaCare should adopt Lean to improve care quality from good to consistently exceptional.

In nearby Brillion, Wisconsin, the Ariens Corporation has been manufacturing rotary tillers for agricultural use since the 1930s. Expanding to lawn-mowing equipment and snow blowers kept the company vital and growing. Ariens first introduced Lean manufacturing principles into its factories in 1998. ThedaCare's experience applying these production-system tools—from its leaders' first visit to Ariens to the widespread engagement with Lean in evidence today at its clinics and hospitals—is described in *On the Mend* by Toussaint and Roger Gerard (2010). ThedaCare, along with Virginia Mason Medical Center, was one of the earliest pioneers in applying Lean to remove waste and improve the quality of healthcare processes.

If doctors today resist incorporating standard work into what they see as the "art" of medicine, in the early years of Lean experiments in healthcare the very idea seemed preposterous. Even applying the *language* of Lean to clinical processes was pushing boundaries and raising ire. Generally speaking, the Lean paradigm doesn't sit very well with most clinicians on first encounter. Especially for physicians, "standard work" translates into an impingement on autonomy.

Direct involvement of physicians in improvement workshops or events is the best remedy for moving beyond that mind-set. Active engagement with the tools that make waste and inefficiency transparent can make converts of cynics. It helps for physicians to visit other healthcare organizations that have had successes benefitting both patients and clinicians. Site visits can help answer physicians' questions and dispel concerns about how approaches used to improve manufacturing can help physicians and patients. But, for pathfinders such as ThedaCare, no health delivery systems at that time offered opportunities for clinicians to see, experience, and learn about Lean.

In the early days, ThedaCare doctors met the Lean transformation with skepticism and apprehension. For doctors used to touching every decision that affects their practice, Lean's team approach left many feeling disenfranchised. Their sense was that they were losing something important to them—their own decision-making prerogative. The Lean consultants had come from manufacturing, where team changes to processes could be made in a more or less top-down fashion. Physicians felt that these consultants may have missed a beat in transferring their previous experiences to healthcare. In recalling those early days, Kathy Franklin, then an internal organizational development (OD) consultant, reported that ThedaCare did amend its approach and began to involve many more physicians on improvement teams and in *kaizen* events to increase their ownership over redesign team results.

Top-Down Changes

The then-wobbly relationship between ThedaCare and its primary care physicians took another hit when, in 2003, ThedaCare announced three changes to the benefit package. Physicians' contribution to their health plan premiums went from 0 to 25 percent; the system's unannounced switch in the medical malpractice policy put the physicians at financial risk for "tail" coverage; and physicians, along with all ThedaCare staff, transitioned from a defined-benefit pension plan to a defined-contribution plan. These major human resources–related changes, made without physician input, sparked outrage. With five-year "out clauses" expiring, what would keep disenfranchised physicians from migrating to other systems or returning to private practice?

Consistency Across the System

Patient-experience data were pointing to the need for consistency. According to Brian Burmeister, then–chief operating officer (COO) of the primary care division, "We could no longer accept that patients would have different experiences depending on what door they walked through." While access and branding were raising the heat for practices to coalesce and function in new ways, tension and acrimony chipped away at mutual trust.

Both the system and the doctors were becoming entrenched in perceptions unhelpful to success. Burmeister remarked, "Then it was time to call the questions: What was reasonable for doctors to expect of the system, and what was the system going to need from its primary care providers?"

RESETTING THE RELATIONSHIP: DIALOGUE AND CLEAR EXPECTATIONS

The benefit changes that exacerbated tensions between the system and doctors did affect the 2004 strategic plan. In that plan, leaders put forth the goal of an improved relationship between employed providers and ThedaCare. Long and Toussaint knew of Jack Silversin's and my work on compacts from Jack's speaking engagements at IHI conferences and other national meetings. Leadership invited Jack to come to Appleton to discuss the process and his potential involvement.

The Process: Forging a New Compact

Establishing Clear Goals
We ask those interested in crafting a new compact the following questions: What's the problem you're trying to solve? What isn't happening that you hope a compact will help make happen?

For this organization, the compact was intended to improve communication, build trust, and support "systemness." Would a compact process help mend the strained relationship between employed doctors and the system? How would clear expectations really help providers? Would this explanation seem like "consultant-speak" when presented to providers? ThedaCare's compact advisory group (CAG) came together to explore these issues. Participating in that group were Burmeister, the physician services division's COO; Long, the division's senior medical director; Dean Gruner, MD, chief medical officer (CMO) and division senior VP; and several providers as primary care representatives. From June to September 2004 the CAG met with Franklin, the OD specialist mentioned earlier, to clarify what a compact process could and could not do for ThedaCare and the primary care providers. Through their internal discussions and phone conferences with Silversin, they identified three objectives for compact work:

+ Improve the communication between parties.
+ Increase the role of providers in decisions that affect them.
+ Clarify the expectations of both parties necessary to meet the goals of the providers and organization.

Taking the Plunge
The CAG and Franklin, with guidance from Silversin, designed a process that would touch as many primary care providers as possible, even though a first draft would be developed by about two dozen people. That fall, at an all-provider meeting to lay the groundwork, leaders presented the idea of the compact and also of a planned retreat to draft the compact.

The two-day retreat took place in early December 2004 at Lambeau Field, home of the Green Bay Packers. Organizing this event in the face of general feelings of mistrust gave real import to the gathering. Meeting at the home of the beloved, championship-winning Packers was viewed as a positive gesture. The CAG selected a true cross section of providers and managers from the practices. In all, about 25 people participated. Wisely, leaders included skeptics who would not be "easy sells," who would push back and ensure minority voices were heard.

As Kathy Franklin said, "The real value is in the process." The Lambeau Field discussions led participants to chart out a new deal—literally. They made a chart with columns labeled "Provider Gives" and "The Organization Gives," using this formulation to establish a reciprocity that a simple give/get dichotomy did not sufficiently capture. According to Kathy Qualheim, MD, associate medical director, the formulation had an inherent fairness that mattered to many. Participants used the same language, as much as possible, for the headings of the tenets under both the Provider and Organization columns because the physicians, in particular, felt expectations for both "sides" should be as similar as possible. (The behavioral expectations under each heading are different depending on whether one is a provider or a formal leader.) This "good for the goose, good for the gander" framework was particularly meaningful for ThedaCare at that moment in its history.

Clear and Inclusive Decision Making

Given how the physician services division had evolved, an important need was to clarify how decisions affecting providers should be made. Specifically, if there were to be a new compact, who would have final say about what it included? The Lambeau Field retreat introduced another tool—fair process—that helped in the compact development and was applied to other corporate-level decisions in the years since the compact work was undertaken.

In a 1997 *Harvard Business Review* article, W. Chan Kim and Renée Mauborgne make three critical points about the human need for fairness in decision-making processes:

- We care about the outcome of a decision-making process and are inclined to act consistently with self-interest.
- We also want procedural justice. When we believe the process is fair, we're likely to accept the outcome. This desire for fairness affects our willingness to engage in change and our trust of those who render decisions.
- Bottom line: "Outcomes matter, but no more than the fairness of the processes that produce them."

Leadership took seriously the need to build decision-making processes that were more inclusive of providers and that would produce outcomes more likely to be seen as just. As a result of the retreat, a commitment was made to apply fair process throughout the compact development process and to foster this approach to decision making where appropriate.

Getting to Trust

One objective of the retreat was to share a common understanding of external conditions and how those shaped the vision statement; another objective was to share perspectives on the internal climate. Silversin facilitated an activity that used decks of playing cards, with each card identifying a common "trust-buster," as a safe way to surface behaviors or traditions inside ThedaCare that eroded trust.

Posted as the number one trust-buster was "inability to follow through on low performers." For Gruner, this was eye-opening: "That powerfully showed me that I wasn't the only one who thought we had an issue with accountability—others shared this concern." Coming out of the retreat, accountability and performance management were seen, along with a new compact, as essential to the system's ability to deliver on its vision.

Deciding Who Is Included in the Compact

Each organization needs to decide for itself who will be covered by its compact. ThedaCare has a long history of employing associate providers and respecting them for their clinical expertise, not using them as assistants to doctors. One of ThedaCare's associate medical directors is a nurse practitioner; one practicing nurse practitioner has a doctorate in nursing. There was enough history of treating associate providers on a par with physicians that their inclusion in the compact seemed natural.

Next Steps

The rest of ThedaCare's process to finalize a compact allowed for input and modifications, guided by fair-process tenets.

Regional Meetings

A few days after the retreat, Long and Toussaint shared the results with the ThedaCare board. In February 2005, they organized half-day regional meetings—with mandatory attendance—so all providers could have input into the compact draft. The script for these sessions mirrored the original retreat agenda:

- Senior leaders presented the case for doing compact work, including metrics on care quality and provider satisfaction.
- Leaders drilled down to challenges facing family medicine across the country.

- Toussaint presented ThedaCare's vision for its future.
- Small groups discussed how a clear compact might support alignment and build trust. Jack Silversin facilitated the debrief.
- Leaders allotted extensive time for review of the draft compact, guided by questions such as: Are these the right areas to focus on to strengthen the relationship between providers and the organization? What's missing? What would you change?
- Participants reviewed the draft compact and suggested changes.
- Leaders closed the session with an overview of fair process and how final decisions about the compact would be made.

The power of the process, according to Toussaint, was the dialogue it provoked. "Given where we were in our development as a system, the compact was important to providers deciding they were 'in' or 'out,'" he notes. In a regional meeting, one physician who had been skeptical announced that the process of developing clarity around roles and responsibilities made him want to be part of the system. Toussaint recalls this as a watershed moment because of the impact of that one doctor's view on others. Then, the doctor was an informal leader whose opinions mattered; today, he has a formal leadership role in the division.

The subsequent ramping up of Lean takes the commitment to involve doctors and staff further and pushes decision making closer to the front lines.

Input, Edits, More Discussion

ThedaCare's CAG examined all the feedback and made changes to the draft; this new version then circled back to senior leadership and to the next all-provider meeting. After additional edits, the revised draft went back to each of the nine call groups[1] (at meetings facilitated by Long) for discussion of the compact's implications and for final input. By September, the leadership council, which represented all the practices and division leadership, approved the final compact. An all-provider meeting to celebrate the compact was held on September 22, 2005—more than a year after the start of the process.

Division COO Burmeister recalls that the compact process and the ultimate document were breakthroughs that allowed trust to be rebuilt. This process was given the necessary time for providers to participate in the changes, to digest them, and to accept a different set of expectations.

Exhibit 4.1 ThedaCare Physicians—ThedaCare Compact

Preamble

Our vision is to be the most sought-after health care partner creating measurable, world-class quality outcomes at the lowest cost. Achieving this vision depends on trusting, collaborative partnerships.

    The foundation of this partnership is a set of clearly defined expectations that are mutually beneficial. ThedaCare and ThedaCare Providers are each responsible to hold themselves and each other accountable to the expectations in this compact. This document serves as a framework of needed behaviors and is intended to be adaptable and to evolve over time. Our dedication to continued dialogue is key to making this compact a valuable and useful set of agreements that support our ability to achieve our vision.

Provider Gives	The Organization Gives
Patient-centered, customer-focused care I will provide exceptional service for our patients by anticipating and exceeding their unique needs, especially in an evolving competitive market.	**Commitment to primary care and collaborative specialty relationships** While valuing all members of the group, we will build ThedaCare's differential value on the primary care provider–patient relationship model.
World class quality I will provide measurable, world class clinical and service quality (≥ 95th percentile performance) that is visible to patients, employers and our communities.	**World class resources** We will invest in the resources and skills necessary to enable providers to have satisfying careers and achieve our vision.
Collaboration and communication I will work toward a common vision by collaborating and communicating effectively with patients, team members, specialists, and all parts of our system.	**Collaboration and communication** We will actively involve our providers in shaping strategic, clinical and operational decisions.
Leadership I will demonstrate leadership through active involvement at the site, call group, and organizational level.	**Leadership** We will demonstrate leadership by setting a vision that reflects our commitment to lead the market through excellence and innovation.

(continued)

Create a positive work environment I will model and create a work environment that is open, trusting, respectful and fulfilling.	**Create a positive work environment** We will model and create a work environment that is open, trusting, respectful and fulfilling.
Flexibility I will seek new solutions and adopt new practices in order to improve my performance.	**Flexibility** We will continuously seek ways to improve how we lead and manage our organization.
Recognition and reward I will recognize and celebrate the accomplishments of the organization and my team members.	**Recognition and reward** We will provide compensation and benefits that reflect the group's accomplishments and enable us to attract and retain the best providers. We will demonstrate appreciation and celebrate provider and team contributions.
Fiscally responsible I will manage resources that ensure the best value for my patients and for the organization and its customers.	**Fiscally responsible** We will deliver the best value—exceptional quality at the lowest cost for our consumers while exceeding financial targets.

Source: ThedaCare. Used with permission.

At the original retreat that initiated ThedaCare's compact work, there was rich discussion about the provider's and ThedaCare's responsibilities. While the key points were distilled to create the compact in Exhibit 4.1, the granularity and specific examples that were part of the discussion were captured in a backup document. In recruiting and other human resources (HR) materials, this document with illustrative behaviors under each heading is appended to the compact. Drilling down one level was never intended to be all-inclusive but instead to flesh out what each key statement in the compact means in practical terms.

Detailed behaviors from each "side" of the compact for one tenet, *Collaboration and communication*, are as follows:

PROVIDER: I will work towards a common vision by collaborating and communicating effectively with patients, team members, specialists, and all parts of our system.

- ◆ Actively listen and share ideas
- ◆ Use available communication methods to seek and give information

- Seek constructive ways to communicate when someone else's behavior is causing a problem
- Enhance communication with specialists to ensure the best care of patients

ORGANIZATION: We will actively involve our providers in shaping strategic, clinical and operational decisions.

- Seek involvement and participation from providers early in the process when business decisions (e.g., marketing, contracting, product design, etc.) impact clinic operations and strategic initiatives
- Actively listen and share ideas
- Use available communication methods to seek and give information
- Communicate emerging strategies, ideas and changes
- Understand, anticipate, and communicate marketplace changes
- Give providers the information they need to be effective in improvement

THEDACARE'S VISION AND LEADERSHIP PHILOSOPHY

To always set and deliver the highest standard of health care performance in measurable and visible ways so our customers are confident they are making the right decision in choosing us.
—*ThedaCare vision statement*

ThedaCare's vision statement continues to be the foundation for its compact work. The compact represents the agreement between the organization and physicians to take actions that bring ThedaCare closer to its vision.

Another facilitator of the compact work is senior leaders' belief in the principles of servant leadership as espoused by Robert Greenleaf (1977, 1998). In the 1990s when he was CMO of the Touchpoint Health Plan, Dean Gruner (now ThedaCare's CEO) read Greenleaf's work. He shared his thinking with ThedaCare Physicians's senior leadership team and call-group leaders. The mind-set that, as a leader, you sit with, listen to, and respect others fits naturally with the compact. In Gruner's words, "It all works together—servant leadership, reciprocal duties expressed as a compact, and our Lean initiatives. All revolve around making issues transparent, getting things in the open, or, in the case of Lean, up on a wall. That leadership philosophy is synergistic with and reinforces what Lean teaches us about management and the values expressed in our compact."

CHANGING ROLES

Since the formation of the division, the ThedaCare physicians leadership council had been tasked with providing input and making decisions on behalf of the division. However, the leadership council was composed of the practice manager and physician leader from each call group—in doctors' eyes, neither had authority over them. They looked to leadership council members solely to ensure that physicians' voices would be heard, not as leaders to whom they were accountable. In most practices, the doctors strove for consensus; everyone sat around the conference table and had a voice in decisions—and all voices were equal. That mind-set didn't necessarily change when practices joined the system.

The compact discussions highlighted the need to do additional work with local physician leadership. It was clear that delegation of meaningful authority to a peer was novel and challenging for those selected for leadership and for everyone else. It meant that the leadership council functioned as an operations group. As the vision for the system became clearer and the imperative for change more obvious, the inability of leadership council members to effectively deal with performance issues and engage providers in change became more apparent.

Altering the Status Quo

Empowering the Leadership Council

Two steps were taken. After finalizing the compact, the leadership council selected a subgroup to develop strategies for more effective communication and coordination between the physician services division and the larger system. The strategy group's purpose was primarily advising system leadership on important issues that had implications for primary care and employed physicians; it met monthly with system leadership for nearly five years. It also regularly met alone for development and education about impending issues and trends so that members could provide meaningful input at the system level.

As another step, leaders addressed the broader issue of legitimate authority so that both practice managers and physician leaders could be more effective locally and, with empowered members, the leadership council could transform into a mature decision-making and strategic governance group for the division. Once the leadership council was more fully empowered and able to be the link with the system, the strategy group was dissolved.

Leadership Development for Physicians

Greg Long and Kathy Franklin took a close look at what it would take for physician leaders to be more effective and feel more successful. The result was a leadership-development program that focused on leading change, performance-related discussions, and coaching for behavioral expectations outlined in the compact. Long recalls one physician leader's response to an invitation to role-play a difficult conversation: "I'd rather have my spleen out than do this." According to Long, "That succinctly captured what many leaders felt then about what we were asking them to do. The role-playing was rated one of the highlights of that session. Participants valued the opportunity to try out difficult conversations in a safe environment. Since then, developing and strengthening their willingness to lead change has been a priority."

"Legitimate Authority"

To be effective, these leaders had to sense that their authority was legitimate and reasonable. The division's leadership council, tasked with defining "legitimate authority," proposed: "Shared responsibility and authority, with the Clinic Administrator, for meeting clinic and call group performance expectations, including provider performance feedback and performance management." They also identified the key competencies they, as a group of clinic administrators and physician leaders, felt were most important for leaders. Using a card-sort activity, they narrowed a list of 67 leadership competencies down to 5:

- Confronting direct reports and others
- Conflict management
- Managerial courage
- Building effective teams
- Managing vision and purpose

These competencies were built into the individual development plans of administrators and physician leaders.

Today, based on their skills and leadership potential, employed-physician leaders are selected by consensus to help ensure appointed leaders are respected by colleagues and seen as having leadership qualities. The leaders are paid an annual stipend that takes into account time away from patient care, the size and scope of the practice for which they're accountable, and recognition for the role itself. Most are compensated 0.1 to 0.2 full-time-equivalent units for this work.

For ThedaCare, strengthening the connection between practices and the system through effective local leadership and clarifying leaders' roles has paid off. Primary care physician turnover in 2013 was under 1 percent. On an Advisory Board Company survey, ThedaCare primary care physicians reported high levels of engagement: 48 percent in the "very engaged" and 41 percent in the "engaged" categories in 2013. In the same year, *Consumer Reports* noted ThedaCare as one of two groups in Wisconsin to earn the highest rating for all but one of seven measures. Wisconsin Collaborative for Healthcare Quality (2014) identified ThedaCare as leading Wisconsin in clinical quality. In addition, *Hospitals & Health Networks* magazine has for ten years named ThedaCare as one of the nation's "most wired" systems.

USES AND LEGACY

As a Guidance Tool

Tina Bettin, APNP, DNP; two medical assistants; and one receptionist are the entire staff at TCP Manawa, ThedaCare's smallest clinic. Bettin participated in the Lambeau Field retreat. She says, "The compact's not a hammer, but if any provider isn't doing what's expected the compact is a great guidance tool for pointing out behaviors it would otherwise be harder to discuss." In her experience, younger providers bring a different twist to the traditional compact. They tend to prioritize work and personal time differently than older colleagues do and want to know more explicitly "what's in it for me?" when asked to take on responsibilities assumed by an earlier generation to be part of citizenship. The compact is a concrete way to state that the organization is asking something of them; that this street is two-way. Bettin also credits the compact with minimizing disparity among clinics that vary in size and complexity. Such systemness was critical to the successful adoption of ThedaCare's new delivery model that builds on the IHI open-access work and standardizes rooming practices across the system.

Clarification for New Hires

ThedaCare's physician recruiter introduces the compact to all primary care physicians considering employment there. Along with the mission, vision, and True North metrics (measures of progress on key strategies), it defines what ThedaCare seeks from employed physicians and helps identify those most likely to fit the ThedaCare ethos. CMO Long believes the low voluntary-turnover rate is in part a function of getting the match right in recent years. Mark Hallett, MD, chief clinical officer, meets with all candidates during their interviews to screen for cultural fit. He explains, "As part of my standardized work, I routinely reference the TCP-ThedaCare compact and describe it as one of the cornerstones of our culture.

In addition, I explain fair process and more recently have added our Values and Behaviors to present a comprehensive picture of the culture here for providers."

Template for Performance Review and Career Development

ThedaCare has built its compact into provider performance–review and career-development processes—both designed to be developmental for providers as well as an annual opportunity for providers to give feedback on how the organization is meeting its commitments. Greg Long began the work of incorporating the compact into the annual review process. This idea was picked up by Hallett, who took performance feedback to the next step, specifically developing a new format and building in leadership accountability that ensured that feedback occurred.

On the first of several forms providers fill out before a review meeting, the compact's "gives" are listed in two columns, with a blank middle column in which providers indicate what's going well and what's not. The form invites providers to comment on their own ability to meet their commitments and to rate ThedaCare's track record in keeping its commitments. This opportunity reinforces the point that all providers at ThedaCare have obligations and are entitled to have expectations of ThedaCare.

In 2012, 93 percent of providers had annual performance reviews using this process.

As a Foundation for a Delivery Model

To create a delivery model that is unmatched in the eyes of our consumers and positions us as a destination employer.
    —*ThedaCare delivery-system mission*

ThedaCare actualizes its patient focus through what it calls its "delivery model"— shorthand for the constellation of system interactions with patients. Implementing the delivery model is standard work for all staff and providers.

The compact's influence is seen in the language and layout of a document that outlines the standards of work—called "commitments to patients"—and what is needed from providers, staff, and administration for the delivery model to be consistently implemented. Specific provider "gives" are spelled out (e.g., time-sensitive in-basket work is completed within two hours of the initial opening of an encounter). The document also lists benefits, or "gets," of following prescribed steps (e.g., more accurate charts lead to better quality and better coding).

Maureen Pistone, senior VP of HR for the system, describes the compact as foundational to the success of the delivery model. What's different about the patient visit in this model? In Maureen's view, "Everything." She continues, "This model changes how medical assistants (MAs) room patients, it changes the order of work for MAs and providers, and it relies on adherence to standard work." She credits the consistency this model has brought to patient visits to the fact that physicians, other providers, and staff built it together with a lot of dialogue. And, after further development, physicians shared it with their peers. Pistone asserts that the decision to use a "give" and "get" framework to outline the expectations would never have happened in the absence of the provider compact.

As a Commitment to Staff

Pistone described another way that compact thinking—clarifying both sides of a deal—has infused the organization. A no-layoff philosophy that goes back to 1988 still stands at ThedaCare. (Lean work could have been sabotaged if redesign had meant that staff would be made redundant.) In 2009, the HR department and managers sat together to draft—and then vet with staff—the Employment Guiding Principles, which describe what ThedaCare and the employee are expected to give in the relationship. As Pistone explains, "We commit to not laying staff off but we're not saying they get to keep their job if it no longer exists. People need to accept development so they can perform a different role or they need to be willing to travel to another site in our system. For our part, we communicate early on if there's to be a role change, and we help each individual find meaningful work." Employee "gives" listed in the document include:

I am dependable, responsible and flexible in how, when and where I work; I am committed to my own growth and development and am willing to learn.

ThedaCare "gives" include:

We provide stable employment and job security; we provide the resources and training for staff to deliver high quality care and personalized customer service, including best practice research and the development of standard work processes.

This explicit compact outlines what's expected of employees in a no-layoff organization while describing how ThedaCare helps employees live up to these expectations.

AN OPEN QUESTION: IS IT TIME FOR THEDACARE TO REVISIT ITS COMPACT?

In the fall of 2013, a number of ThedaCare leaders and providers I interviewed saw the compact as very much alive, describing its usefulness in performance-related conversations. Others suggested that the compact's visibility had faded and that, given its value to the organization, it should be revisited. One doctor said that while it's not at the top of his mind, the compact functions for him like an insurance policy—it's there for him to reference if he feels leaders are violating some compact tenet. It facilitates a conversation when what's happening—or not happening—is outside the compact. Another physician who didn't give the compact any thought on a day-to-day basis said that she trusts ThedaCare to solicit provider input, in part because doing so is part of the compact and is now routine. She reported, "Even if I'm not at the table, I know that some physician is."

ThedaCare is growing again by acquiring specialty practices. Given this and other changes since the compact work was done nearly a decade ago, system leadership is asking: Do we refresh the compact we have and bring specialists into this deal? Should an employed specialist compact look different? And, should we have clearer expectations of those medical staff who are independent and will remain so? If we do refresh the compact, should we design a comprehensive input process, as in the past, or can a scaled-back project accomplish our ends?

Reflecting the original need the compact was meant to address, it has been used almost exclusively to *build the relationship between individual practitioners and the system*. Relationships *among* providers aren't the focus for either leaders or providers when they think about the compact. If they refresh the compact, should they consider the extent to which it fosters interdependence among providers? In the new world of accountable care organizations (ACOs), integration and care coordination will be critical to success—making effective collaboration among all parts of the ACO a top priority. Can the compact help with that challenge?

One leader reported that ThedaCare's PDSA (plan-do-study-act) mentality— the bedrock of its Lean work—would suggest that the compact should be routinely scrutinized to determine how it could be improved. To this leader, doing so is consistent with the improvement mind-set prevalent at ThedaCare.

SUMMING UP

The compact process had a fundamental impact on the system: It moved providers from a "me" to a "we" mentality. The level of connection between individual primary care providers and the system is now strong. ThedaCare's compact work, done nearly ten years ago, healed a rift and helped the system leverage its potential to coordinate care and provide outstanding quality.

Since then, the trend toward physician employment has surged (Kane and Emmons 2013). In the past five years, hospital purchases of physician practices have risen 30 to 40 percent (Kavilanz 2013). Looking at this reality, ThedaCare's compact process offers several key lessons that other organizations can benefit from:

- *The timing was right; and many felt that the lack of trust was unsustainable.* The time was ripe for honest conversation. While doctors cite both the sale of the health plan and changed HR policies as the proverbial straws that did the camel in, unclear expectations for over ten years had already taken a toll. With local leaders able to function only as advocates for their clinics' needs, the system was hampered. When doctors exercised their option to exit the system, leadership had to pay attention. This confluence of issues made it an opportune time for the honest dialogue that proved to be healing.
- *Leaders committed to look at their behavior and change.* The authentic commitment of leadership, and their integrity, also played a significant role. Despite their frustrations, physicians understood that leaders genuinely wanted to be constructive and to improve relationships with providers. In Greg Long, the compact work had a visible sponsor who was totally committed to a full airing of issues. John Toussaint and Dean Gruner signaled the system's support by being at the retreat and at the regional all-provider compact meetings.
- *ThedaCare has bench strength.* ThedaCare had the expertise to help design a thoughtful compact process and then to develop local leadership talent. Every step of the work was supported by ThedaCare's OD professionals. Not every organization of this size has such sophisticated organizational development staff. With this in-house capability, the external consultant (Silversin) was used appropriately—to lend authority and perspective. Leaders took responsibility and did not look to an outsider to carry their messages. The more that an organization can do on its own, the more it owns the process and the outcomes.

NOTE

1. The 27 clinics are split into 9 call groups that allow geographically proximate physicians to share the burden of calls.

CHAPTER 5

Stillwater Medical Group: A Multispecialty Group Affirms Interdependence Before a Hospital Merger

STILLWATER MEDICAL GROUP

Stillwater is one of the oldest towns in Minnesota. Today part of the Twin Cities metro area, in the late 1830s it was the first outpost of settlers in the St. Croix River valley. The lucrative lumber trade that plied the St. Croix River brought prosperity to Stillwater; wives of lumber barons funded the predecessor to the modern Lakeview Hospital. Many in Stillwater take pride in their city's place in Minnesota history. The leaders of Stillwater Medical Group (SMG) say that this local reputation for being "first in the state" is a major reason for the organization's drive to excel.

In 2005, SMG created a compact that still adds value even though the group is now part of a large system, Minneapolis-based HealthPartners. When its compact work began, SMG was wrestling with the question of how to adapt to economic pressures in a changing healthcare landscape. When remaining an independent medical group did not seem feasible, the group began getting its own house in order as part of a merger process. To strengthen their own group ethos, SMG's leaders and physicians designed a compact they call their "internal declaration of interdependence." This group practice's commitment to its compact has helped it to be a respected partner to local Lakeview Hospital and still helps the physicians maintain their core identity while contributing to the larger system of which they are a part.

A TIME OF TRANSITION

Between 2003 and 2005, the need for change became increasingly apparent for SMG. According to Steve Scallon, MD, "There was a feeling among physician leadership that we really could be better together in many ways."

Scallon was a board member when the group's performance data indicated things weren't as good as assumed. The group's publicly reported quality metrics relating to chronic conditions such as diabetes were lower than the community average. It was also becoming clear that unprecedented capital needs were looming; the facility needed repairs, significant expansion, and modernizing; and IT systems were outdated at a time when moving to electronic medical records was inescapable. All this occurred after a period when some physicians' salaries had fluctuated enough to capture their attention. While there was no single catalyst, a number of issues converged and a general sense that change was needed reverberated throughout the group. The leadership began serious talks about partnering with Lakeview Hospital.

Merging wasn't a novel idea; some conversations with Lakeview had taken place five years earlier. At that earlier point, the timing didn't feel right. However, by 2005 the hospital and the clinic wanted to build a wider regional presence; there was interest in attracting specialists just when income stability and capital needs were on SMG's radar screen. Leaders began to have serious discussions. Any merger would mean that SMG's physicians would step away from their status as owners of a partnership to being employees of a not-for-profit system. As SMG's merger with the hospital seemed a likely outcome of discussions, the idea of an explicit compact between the clinic's physicians and SMG became more relevant.

With 50 practicing physicians, the old culture that emphasized physician autonomy was increasingly problematic—even if economics had allowed the group to retain its independent status. Leaders saw a link between the slow spread of quality initiatives and each doctor's prerogative to practice as he or she saw fit. Despite the effort that SMG was putting into care-improvement projects, physicians felt entitled to opt out of any change not to their liking. All doctors still customized their own daily schedules to fit their individual preferences. Autonomy even had an impact on the group's ability to effectively formulate and carry out any strategy; any one doctor could call an end to discussions, and all doctors retained the prerogative to say "no" to any decisions they did not make.

In addition, SMG leaders could see that being a reliable and trusted part of an integrated system was critical to the group's being treated as such. Lakeview was not interested in "taking over." Early talks clarified that, in any new entity, both the hospital and the group would maintain their own integrity; each would have a board, whose members would sit on a larger, system-level board. But for SMG to be an effective partner with the hospital, leaders felt the group had to evolve, that all doctors had to act in the best interest of the whole organization or the hospital would have little choice but to steer with a firm and visible hand.

Five years earlier, a significant transition in governance had taken place: the board's size was reduced and representatives were elected. At SMG, every partner physician had sat on the board. In deciding to elect representatives, SMG took the first step toward a more mature governance structure. By the time of the merger discussions, the SMG management committee members had begun to see themselves less as representatives of constituencies—advocates for particular departments—and more as members of a body governing the whole.

When the idea of the compact surfaced in a learning collaborative, Charlie Hipp, MD, then the group's president, seized on it as a way to more broadly engage doctors and staff in ongoing quality improvement, to up the group's game relative to quality, and to help doctors transition to being responsible members in a new organizational structure. It was a way to prepare the physicians to no longer be owners and to bring a new relationship to life; doctors, he felt, had obligations to the group and the group had obligations to them.

A LEARNING COLLABORATIVE DESIGNED TO CHANGE GROUP CULTURE

SMG had been a longtime participant in care-improvement learning activities sponsored by the Minneapolis-based Institute for Clinical Systems Improvement (ICSI). ICSI was founded by HealthPartners Health Plan and several local medical groups to convene experts to develop best-practice guidelines to prevent, diagnose, and treat common health conditions. From these beginnings in 1993, the organization expanded to include most group practices across Minnesota. Additional nonprofit insurers and health plans in Minnesota and Wisconsin signed on to create, with the medical groups, a unique laboratory to advance evidence-based care and to test other improvement ideas. Between 2004 and 2010, ICSI offered its medical group members the opportunity to learn about culture change as it relates to quality improvement through a collaborative workshop, Leading a Culture of Quality (LCQ).

LCQ built on the successful model of ICSI's other collaboratives. This offering supported participating groups to learn about culture change through periodic meetings, conference calls, and assignments geared to assess norms or take actions to shape a culture more aligned with care improvement. A shortcoming of approaches that involve some staff members taking time off to hone process-improvement skills or learn about the latest evidence-based practices is that these individuals then try to implement—in an old culture—new and better ways of working. ICSI, however, offered this series of workshops and related assignments as a chance to directly address the widespread issue of cultural impediments to sustained improvement.

Jack Silversin and I served as faculty for this ICSI collaborative, and our ideas and approaches were woven into the curriculum.

SMG was one of the first organizations to commit to LCQ. Stillwater signed on, according to Hipp, "Because we had already been thinking along these lines; it wasn't a big stretch for us. Embedding a continuous-improvement mentality into the organization was appealing." Along with Hipp, Larry Morrissey, who was then the medical director, was convinced of two things: SMG needed to move from projects to culture change, and it had to more broadly engage doctors and staff—improvement couldn't be the purview of just a few. At the LCQ collaborative, the team from SMG first encountered the compact as a way to shift culture.

LEADERS GO FIRST

A truth I've come to deeply appreciate over the years is that when an organization asks its physicians to change, their leaders have to "go first." Leaders have to cross the bridge first before being able to mobilize others to do likewise. The success of SMG's compact work hinges in no small part on the investment its leaders made in understanding the limits of their current culture and how a different compact would affect their own work. If they were going to take the group in a new direction, they wanted to be on solid ground and be clear about what they would be asking of colleagues.

A milestone was a bus trip to St. Cloud, Minnesota, that SMG leaders had taken to meet with physician colleagues who had just completed a medical practice–hospital merger. Hipp and Morrissey recalled the journey home from the meeting, which allowed all those on the bus to process what they had learned. The ride-home debate helped that group clarify what SMG needed to do to ensure a successful future. One salient conclusion was that a mind-set shift among SMG doctors was imperative, especially as it related to decision making. Relying on consensus to decide major issues—such as changes in the compensation formula—would be a liability in the rapidly changing healthcare landscape. The individuals on the bus concluded that the old way would not work anymore, but they had no clear view of what the new way should be.

Leaders saw the compact—which they were learning about in the LCQ collaborative—as a framework to introduce the kind of changes they felt the group needed to make. Hipp reported, "This was not a simple turn-on-the-light-switch process. First the executive committee of the board [these individuals had participated in the LCQ collaborative meetings] had to wrestle with how a compact could and could not help." These conversations continued for months and included critiques of the early drafts of what, eventually, would become the compact. Each proposed tenet was vetted and compared to the currently operating compact. The choice of words and behavioral examples were given time and attention. Each proposed element was examined through the lens of, "Why should this element be included?"

These meetings proved to be significant in developing the leaders' ownership of the need to change and their commitment to the compact as a tool in that process. This investment by leaders pays dividends at the stage when ideas are widely shared and physicians push back. Firm commitment to what they had debated and clarified helped SMG leaders gain the courage to marshal the group around adaptive changes (discussed in Chapter 1). "Adaptive change" is Ronald Heifetz's term for a change that threatens long-standing habits, beliefs, or traditions; a change that provokes anger, frustration, and feelings of loss.

During the run-up to the compact and to the merger with Lakeview, the board occasionally held meetings off-site so participants would be removed from the exigencies of the practice and have space to reflect and plan. They read and discussed leadership books as a group, starting with Jim Collins's *Good to Great* (2001). It was another investment that prepared them to "cross the bridge first."

DECLARING INTERDEPENDENCE

In the management committee meetings, a compact draft began taking shape. The leaders always viewed the compact as embodying a common understanding about the gives and gets in the relationship between providers and the group; it was never considered a contract in the legal sense. At one point, the director of human resources, Carol Nagele-Vitalis, suggested the document focus on "interdependence," which immediately resonated with others. At SMG the compact includes the group's advanced practice providers—physician assistants and nurse practitioners; thus, technically, it's a provider compact. The organization's "gives" were defined as responsibilities of the practice administrator, president, and executive committee.

Over several months, the management committee vetted the idea of the compact at periodic all-provider meetings. (To make these meetings as productive as possible, Hipp and other leaders would meet ahead of time with individuals they predicted would contribute negativity to discussions that needed to be candid.) At these meetings, leaders shared their thinking about why a compact would help and what it could include. Input was woven into "The Declaration of Interdependence" (Exhibit 5.1).

The watershed of the process was an evening meeting of all providers in late 2005. Jack Silversin, on-site to work with the effort's leaders, also participated in

Exhibit 5.1 Stillwater Medical Group Provider Compact

"The Declaration of Interdependence"
Provider Gives:
◆ Provide patient-centered care and service
◆ Be flexible, willing to change and open to innovation
◆ Be on the team, not above or outside
◆ Stay informed and actively involved
◆ Recognize and support organizational leadership
◆ Be accountable for personal and group results
◆ Be a good steward of organizational and healthcare resources
Stillwater Medical Group Gives:
◆ Provider-directed group practice
◆ Engagement in decision making and fair process
◆ Organizational support and resources to practice best medicine
◆ Fair compensation based on market and group performance
◆ Excellent communication

Source: Stillwater Medical Group. Used with permission.

this meeting. He had met separately with the clinic management committee just prior to the start of the session and suggested that the leaders take seats at the front of the room to demonstrate their solidarity with regard to the issues to be discussed.

The evening's objectives were to get all providers engaged in conversations about quality, upcoming capital needs, and the implications of merging with the hospital and of developing a compact. At the start of the meeting, Morrissey declared, "We're not as good as we think we are." Asking Silversin to present his observations—about what was changing for medical groups and how the traditional physician compact can be a barrier to future success—lent credibility to the leaders' call for change. Morrissey reported that having an outsider deliver this message resulted in broad acceptance by physicians, rather than challenge. The conversations, while not always easy, set a tone of openness.

The proposed compact was printed and used as a visual aid for the main presentation. Each leader stood up and talked about his commitment to the compact, and each signed it. Then, in a rather impromptu move, other providers who wanted to add their signatures were invited to do so. All doctors except one (who later left the group) lined up to sign the compact. Those who led the effort were surprised at the others' receptivity to the compact and the voluntary signing. Those actions indicated openness to being a new kind of medical group: one in which group interests and performance trumped personal preferences. Recalling those consequential events, Hipp said, "I'll always remember that night."

After the compact was signed, the three key physician leaders—Scallon, Hipp, and Morrissey—and the practice administrator continued meeting with groups of eight to ten providers to give them a chance to ask questions, challenge ideas, and more thoroughly understand why the compact was the way forward. These meetings were the start of implementation. They communicated that this was not a passing fad, but that everyone was expected to live up to the agreement they had signed.

A LIVING DOCUMENT

In a few years, the signatures on the large-format compact soaked into the foam-core board and faded into illegibility. When a slight modification was made to improve the compact, the new version was mounted on a different medium, which the providers re-signed.

The large-format, signed Declaration of Interdependence is in the administrative office of the group president, Andy Dorwart, MD. The president's role has grown in importance since the start of the compact work and as the group partnered first with the hospital and now with HealthPartners; what had been a one-quarter-time position now is three-quarters' time. The CEO appoints the president, with the consent of the management committee, which also is now appointed rather than elected.

Using the Compact

At SMG, the compact has not been static; additions reflect new imperatives or changed circumstances. One provider responsibility was added regarding resource stewardship; the new wording better reflects the organization's commitment to the triple aim of quality care, population health, and patient experience.

Hiring and New Hires

Dorwart uses the compact during interviews with every physician who visits SMG with an interest in joining the group. To him, "Successful recruitment and retention comes down to fit. It's far easier for us to hire someone who fits our culture than to separate someone who's not working out. Severing doctor–patient relationships is difficult and can risk the reputation of the group." From interviewees, Dorwart has received feedback that SMG spends more time than other organizations in up-front discussions of cultural fit.

At orientation, every new provider gets a copy of the compact and is asked to sign the large-format version. The department chair and administrator also discuss the compact with new hires in their first meeting. Dorwart believes the compact is more valuable in shaping physician behavior than mission, vision, or values historically have been. The SMG compact signals that the group has high expectations of its provider members. The subtext is that providers have unique roles and special responsibilities (not extra privileges). Dorwart has seen other compacts with many more "promises" but believes that the more promises made, the greater the opportunity for individuals to drift away from those promises. If management or providers are held accountable for only some of the tenets, the meaningfulness of the compact as a whole fades. Its utility to shape culture is minimized.

Performance-Related Discussions

The support a compact can provide to physician leaders at all levels deserves comment. An explicit compact is worth the time and effort to develop even if it only helps doctor leaders to begin performance-related conversations. Hipp notes, "I was grateful to have the compact when I was president and it was my responsibility to have performance-related conversations with physicians." When behavior inconsistent with the compact continues, physicians have been asked to agree to performance-improvement plans.

Most physician leaders feel they are on shaky ground when talking to another doctor about his or her behavior unless the behavior is obviously egregious—in which case, most leaders will step up. More difficult are conversations about inappropriate behavior that has an impact on other doctors or staff, involves potential harm, or reflects badly on the institution, but that isn't close to grounds for dismissal. If all a leader can fall back on is "That's not how we do things around here," things can easily go off track. A compact that doctors themselves helped craft is a platform for a different conversation—giving the initiator firm ground on which to stand. One doctor leader said the compact erases much of the anxiety he would otherwise have during performance-related conversations: "It's not personal—this isn't me imposing my values on you. The compact is what you agreed to do as a condition of being here."

Letting a Physician Go

The compact has also been useful when a doctor has to be separated from the group. Dorwart views those occasions this way: "I'm not letting anyone go; you are choosing to not be here by not accepting policy or the compact." It is doctors' responsibility to abide by group norms; not doing so is viewed as an active and conscious choice.

Fair Process

SMG's compact includes a commitment to use fair process. In practical terms, this has meant that administrators and physician leaders want providers to know that the latter's views are heard. When asked to weigh in on key decisions, physicians are given information so they know what leadership knows. Leaders then have an obligation to listen to what doctors and others believe is important. In choosing an architectural firm to build a new main facility, this process was followed. Fair process resulted in providers and staff saying what was important to them in the new physical space and supported the selected firm in designing an inviting and healing environment without delays, squabble, or rework.

A Shift in Mind-Set

Some people at SMG have had difficulty making the shift to the world the compact represents. Despite the fact that the group kept the compact alive and moved forward with patient-centered care, there are still pockets of "old thinking." Even though such inconsistencies exist, Dorwart proudly points to what he considers a notable success. "Doctors see themselves (and can be held accountable) for being 'on' the team, not above it. This shift in both mind-set and actual behavior is attributed to our compact."

THE PAST, THE PRESENT . . . AND THE FUTURE

In 2011 the Lakeview system partnership with HealthPartners came to fruition. As a result, physicians, in fact, have less opportunity for input. Much more physician input was sought when the group merged with the hospital in 2005. Then, the question on the table was, "Do you want to go in this direction?" Around the HealthPartners integration, physicians' degree of influence was more limited but they were still involved. The framing for provider involvement was more along the lines of: "This is the direction we're going. How do we get to this destination?"

Between 2008 and 2010, the organization made a concerted effort to put patients at the center of care processes and has been able to move ahead successfully with shared decision making. According to then–medical director Morrissey, "The compact allowed this group to make a lot of changes over the eight years since its adoption. I believe what's been achieved is in no small part because of the environment the compact set up." Accomplishments to which the compact work contributed, in his view and that of other leaders, include the following:

- Physicians and providers were open to adoption of a new "care-model process" built on Lean principles. The care model standardizes workflows to allow everyone to function to the highest level of their licensure. For example, pre-visit planning is done by medical assistants, who review needed labs and tests as part of chronic disease or preventative services and order them for the physician to co-sign. There are standardized workflows for all elements of a visit and for the flow of information such as test results. With care-model process champions who include medical, nursing, and operational leaders, this new way of working has been adopted and there is continued commitment to hardwiring it.
- SMG was one of 11 demonstration sites funded by the Informed Medical Decisions Foundation. This funding ran for three years and was extended for an additional two. Morrissey, who championed the informed-decision work, described it as successful in multiple departments in the clinic.
- Patient satisfaction data are tracked with the Consumer Assessment of Healthcare Providers and Systems survey. The leadership wanted SMG to be a leader in Minnesota, and when data showed the organization was not, the compact supported greater transparency in sharing of results with the aim of improving scores. Providers see their own patient-experience scores and the department's overall score. Comments from patients are also shared, along with suggested action steps for improvement, such as "shadow coaching."
- Publicly reported quality measures are "unblinded." The results of work on conditions such as diabetes and asthma are shared with the teams, and data on individual performance on operational metrics are posted. SMG's numbers have consistently improved and are now above average for most of the relevant measures.

Having the compact supports a strong sense of teamwork and openness to innovation. In the years since it was adopted and through all the organizational changes, the prevailing mind-set has been one of putting the group before individual needs and practicing patient-centered care. There's been no backpedaling to an individualistic mind-set. The compact still functions as a tangible reminder that "We are in this together."

Morrissey shared an incident that, to him, sums up the meaning of the compact at SMG. During a discussion about whether it was worthwhile for her to participate in the development of staff standards of behavior, one medical assistant had said, "We're watching to see if the compact will be just a picture on the wall or will lead to providers doing things differently."

The reality is that doctors *are* leaders who, whether or not they are conscious of it, are role models for everyone else in the practice. Morrissey remarked, "When doctors live up to values in the compact, everyone's skepticism toward change diminishes. When doctors change, it matters to everyone who's watching."

Stillwater Medical Group Employees Translate Values into Behaviors

The culture change at SMG "did start with the providers' clarifying their gives and gets," according to Susan Wright, director of primary care operations. A separate effort was undertaken with all other staff to help shift to what Wright calls a "culture of accountability."

Wright and the human resources director felt that a more useful approach than developing a compact would be to turn the group's existing values statement into a statement enumerating specific behaviors that could become standards to which staff commit. They designed a process that enabled staff members to suggest the behaviors. Wright says, "One surprise for me was that staff identified behaviors for standards that are tougher or reach higher than what I and other leaders would have come up with."

Having a provider compact can trigger general culture change. Staff members view physicians as leaders, especially in a group that is physician-owned. For that reason, if staff members don't see those providers as particularly patient-centered, they naturally conclude that patients' needs aren't much of a priority. And while a physician or provider compact can reset expectations of an important segment of the organization, it isn't—in and of itself—enough for cultural transformation across all occupational subcultures.

Determined Action on Values

Wright and others sought to close the gap between the actions of staff and the stated values of the medical group. The group's core values—familiar to anyone working in healthcare—are compassion, accountability, integrity, collaboration, pursuit of excellence, and determination to put patients at the center of all efforts. Most medical organizations espouse these principles. But SMG took the critical step of moving from "great brochure copy" to pinpointing specific behaviors that have translated into quality care and high organizational performance.

The process began with the values. Wright and her co-leader invited the union stewards and representatives from each business area to be part of a working group to brainstorm behaviors that expressed each of the six core values mentioned earlier. Leaders prompted the discussion by asking what individuals personally thought each value meant, and took notes.

As a next step, leaders met with small groups of about eight staff members to further define behaviors. Leaders posted the six values on a wall and asked participants to match each brainstormed behavior with the value it exemplified. Participants could also add behaviors not already considered. The small groups had rich conversations around the meanings of the values and the specific behaviors. Small-group engagement sessions were repeated until every staff member had been involved. The conversations were put in the context of accountability; a good deal of discussion centered on what should happen after the behaviors were written down. A draft document reflecting the work done by all the small groups was circulated for additional feedback. The executive committee of the medical group approved the final version: "Standards of Behavior; written by employees of SMG."

This text remains a living document with meaning and purpose, even though the medical group and the local hospital are branded as Lakeview Health and today are part of the Minneapolis-based HealthPartners System. Staff performance reviews are based on these standards, as are merit increases. Coaching is provided if anyone isn't sure what the standard means for a particular job. Terminations from Lakeview in recent years generally have been related to a breach of expected behavior (as opposed to a skill deficit). A significant part of the interview process of any employee, and more so for any leader, focuses on the standards. The message is, "If these don't match with who you are, you're not going to work out here." Training in accountability, with an emphasis on affirmation and positive acknowledgment, is given to all leaders. Any coaching a leader provides to staff is based on data or actual experience. Performance reviews are viewed as fair and consistent.

Deepening the culture of accountability rests on meeting the needs of the staff, who have set a high bar for what they expect from themselves and others. In Wright's words, "Our employees created the culture they want to work in." Accountability and respect are two sides of the same coin. To not insist staff meet standards that they themselves generated would be disrespectful. As a result of the creation and fair application of the standards of behavior, employees saw less need for union representation, and one union withdrew its petition to represent the SMG staff. With a stronger sense of fair play based on staff-generated standards, employees felt that benefits would not outweigh the cost of belonging to the union.

Instead of a compact that highlights a different relationship, a transformation among staff came from asking them to identify specific behaviors that would give life to values they saw as worthy and important (Exhibit 5.2). By having staff define the standards, not only were clarity, consistency, and accountability achieved, but ownership and deep pride were as well. With all the talk of care improvement, this organization has found that the focus on accountability based on clear standards allows significant gains to be made. Wright feels, "This is our base. When other medical groups ask about our results, I always tell them: Without the bedrock of accountability, you can't get where you really want to go."

Exhibit 5.2 Excerpt from Stillwater Medical Group Employee-Generated Standards of Behavior

Value	Standard of Behavior—Examples
Patient Centered	I will . . . ◆ ask, "What is in the best interest of the patient/family?" ◆ create a lasting impression with a helpful and caring attitude.
Compassion	I will . . . ◆ provide extra comfort and reassurance to exceed my customers' expectations. ◆ treat everyone with dignity and respect, understanding I do not have to like someone to treat them respectfully.
Accountability	I will . . . ◆ choose to have a positive attitude. ◆ own my own mistakes rather than blame someone or something else.
Integrity	I will . . . ◆ "do the right thing" even when no one is looking. ◆ act consistent with my words and "walk the talk."
Collaboration	I will . . . ◆ be ready to help even before I am asked. ◆ recognize our dependence on each other to exceed our patients' expectations.
Pursuit of Excellence	I will. . . ◆ be consistent in the work I do, always working to the best of my ability. ◆ take advantage of opportunities to learn new skills.

Source: Generated originally by staff at Stillwater Medical Group, which later merged with Lakeview Hospital to form Lakeview Health, this document is a living, working tool for all employees at Lakeview Health.

SUMMING UP

The compact has helped SMG maintain a sense of group identity and integrity through significant changes—the growth from about 50 providers to almost 100 in eight years, and Lakeview Health System's merger with HealthPartners. The compact is the tool most often cited as responsible for the group's current cohesion and openness to innovation. Key takeaways from SMG's experience include the following:

- Leaders devoted considerable time to developing their own understanding of market changes, of limitations of the old governance model, and of how an explicit compact could help the group. They met on their own time to read and discuss management concepts; several attended the multiyear program that LCQ became. Their investment strengthened their will and courage to transform an "autonomy–protection–entitlement" mind-set to one in which individuals appreciate the reciprocity of obligations and work for the good of the whole.
- Leaders also worked to ensure every provider understood the compact, holding numerous small-group meetings.
- This is an example of a physician-led process, not one in which an administrator brings the idea to physicians. From the start, physicians were on board and largely generated interest in the compact. A key insight shared by Morrissey is that it would have been damaging if the compact were seen as a way to try to control doctors.
- SMG struck the right balance between employing outside help and relying on its own leaders to explain the concept and get reactions. By participating in the ICSI collaborative (LCQ), the team had a source of support and could get its ideas affirmed. Leaders judiciously used Silversin to present the big picture and explain how the compact has been helpful to other physician groups. Silversin also advised the board. However, the "heavy lifting" of small-group sessions and reworking the draft to capture resonant language was done in-house. Leaders' extensive preparation gave them the courage and skills to have conversations that, especially early in the process, were challenging. Their willingness to directly engage colleagues in conversation was an important key to this group's success with their compact.

CHAPTER 6

Memorial Hermann Physician Network: A Clinically Integrated, Virtual Medical Group

WIDELY DISPERSED, INDEPENDENT-MINDED PHYSICIANS

Memorial Hermann Physician Network (MHMD), a sprawling network of community, academic, and employed doctors that partners with the nine-hospital Memorial Hermann Health System, is a "Texas-sized" independent physician association (IPA). That is to say, its size is distinctive: MHMD covers an extensive geographic area and has a membership that dwarfs that of most physician organizations. With four thousand physicians in the greater Houston area, it is the largest physician network in Texas.

Although the independent doctors in the IPA, who make up the majority of members, value the autonomy of private practice, they also enjoy the teamwork necessary to provide the highest quality of care for their patients. One doctor summed it up like this: "Independence is a way to maintain autonomy and control over my business, set the rules for this practice, and hire those who work for me." Those are powerful motivators for doctors to want to remain independent.

Nearly half of the physicians in the MHMD network participate in Memorial Hermann's highly successful clinical integration (CI) program. CI members determine the quality, safety, and efficiency protocols, which are then implemented throughout their practices and the nine-hospital system. (Memorial Hermann and its network of physicians have earned widespread recognition in these three areas.[1]) The physicians' participation in CI gives them a voice in how they will practice in the future and makes them eligible for bonus pools and performance-based contracts negotiated by the Memorial Hermann Health System (MHHS) and MHMD. MHMD's achievements in physician–hospital alignment, quality, and safety are especially remarkable given that the doctors are largely community-based in small offices ("onesies" and "twosies").

Even in states where physician employment is possible and common, physician–hospital alignment can be an executive's greatest challenge. Close alignment and cooperation are especially critical as reimbursement evolves from fee-for-service to value-based and population management–based models. If physician satisfaction with hospitals is a correlate of loyalty, MHMD is in good standing. The 2012 physician survey conducted by HealthStream Research found 54 percent of physicians were "very satisfied" and 40 percent "satisfied" with Memorial Hermann hospitals—94 percent reporting the top two satisfaction levels is evidence that this system and its medical staff are on the same page.

MHMD's story involves issues of interest to many physician organizations and hospitals. How has this extensive hospital system developed and sustained collaboration with doctors not on the payroll? How does it achieve its impressive quality results? How are explicit, co-developed, reciprocal expectations used to coalesce the membership? What kind of leadership fosters constructive partnerships? Isn't the alignment a result of CI's rewarding physicians out of shared savings? And if a vast network of doctors can partner with a large hospital system, why can't others build the same cooperative spirit and reap benefits for patients, the community, and the doctors?

A LOOK BACK: UNEXCEPTIONAL BEGINNINGS

The roots of MHMD reach back to 1983, when Memorial Health System formed a wholly owned subsidiary—Memorial Hermann Health Network Providers (MHHNP)—to serve employees enrolled in the system's health plan. For close to 20 years this IPA, with about 2,000 physician members, was purely a vehicle for managed-care contracting. Richard Blakely, MD, who was MHMD's chief medical officer for more than 10 years, described the early days as follows: "The best metaphor for the first 20 years or so of the IPA's existence would be physicians as passengers on a cruise ship; they were on board for one, self-centered purpose—to get reasonable contracts. They did not go out of their way to work together to control costs or affect care quality."

That account could easily describe many physician networks at that time.

The Federal Trade Commission and Department of Justice Weigh In

The antitrust threat represented by such networks—negotiating as one body without financial or clinical integration—was not lost on the Federal Trade Commission

(FTC) or the Department of Justice. In 1996 they revised guidelines on how such networks should negotiate contracts (US Department of Justice and Federal Trade Commission 1996). Both agencies continued to scrutinize IPAs, charging a number of provider networks with price-fixing and violations of the new regulations. In 2003 the FTC charged MHHNP with colluding to obtain higher doctor's fees from insurers, thereby driving up healthcare costs in the Houston market. MHHNP settled, admitting no violations, and a consent decree barred it from some previous actions on physicians' behalf. It could negotiate only if specific criteria were met, which related to doctors' working together for efficiency and quality.

A 2002 FTC ruling related to two Denver-area physician organizations granted physicians the ability to contract together as long as they were participants in a "qualified risk-sharing joint arrangement" or a "qualified clinically integrated joint arrangement." To be a qualified clinically integrated joint arrangement:

1. physician members must "participate in active and ongoing programs to evaluate and modify their clinical practice patterns, creating a high degree of interdependence and cooperation among physicians in order to control costs and ensure the quality of services provided"; and
2. with regard to reimbursement or other conditions, the entity has to make significant efficiencies through the joint arrangement (Federal Trade Commission 2014).

The FTC held that no action would be taken against organizations that meet the threshold for creating efficiencies while not driving out competition (Simon, Brooks, and Rossman 2009), thereby establishing the legal basis for clinically integrated physician networks. The game-changing nature of the ruling lies in its requiring independent doctors to create "a high degree of interdependence and cooperation among physicians in order to control costs and ensure the quality of services provided" (Federal Trade Commission 2014). In some traditional group practices—where doctors practice under one roof—acknowledged interdependence and collaboration to control costs and improve quality are still elusive.

With its 2004 FTC settlement, MHHNP was "grounded" as a vehicle for contracting jointly on behalf of its physician members. However, the settlement did not prohibit the Houston-area physicians from continuing as a clinically integrated organization. But if they chose that option, physicians would need to embrace the role of all-hands-on-deck quality champions—working *together* to improve care and reduce costs. The news that the old arrangement was over engendered bad feelings among doctors. Ultimately, however, the ruling breathed life into the IPA and fostered new ways for those in the network to work collectively; to partner with the Memorial Hermann hospitals to raise care quality and reduce costs; and to develop a collaborative esprit among the wide network of community, employed, and academic doctors.

Recognizing Weaknesses

In 2000, Ernst and Young advisors were engaged to examine the business model from a system perspective. One conclusion was that quality, efficiency, safety, and the bottom line would improve if the system functioned *in fact* like a system. The hospitals, the advisors noted, were operating much as independent entities: The nine medical executive committees (MECs) "did their own thing" and each hospital had its own policies. There were fifteen thousand drugs in the formulary. As a management philosophy, "let every flower bloom" was choking the garden—working against leveraging the scale of the system for efficiency.

Doctor engagement had to increase considerably for the system to be more efficient. The first initiative was to ask network physicians to form committees to develop a system-wide formulary. The expectation that committee members would take recommendations back to their hospital's MEC proved unrealistic; committee members weren't necessarily MEC members or leaders in their hospitals. With no mechanism for accountability, recommendations didn't go far.

MOVING TOWARD SYSTEMNESS

It was obvious that hospitals would save money and the system would benefit from having a single formulary and uniform standards. But what was the value proposition for network doctors? As long as MHHNP was set up as a traditional network, no opportunities existed for upside gains for individual doctors.

A journey to Chicago in 2005 was pivotal. On that trip, MHHNP's network CEO Scott Fenn, chief medical officer (CMO) Blakely, and Keith Fernandez, MD, learned how Advocate Physician Partners had implemented a successful CI program among its four thousand members. They proposed that the Memorial Hermann system support a similar program. Blakely reported, "The basic logic of CI felt right to the system leadership: independent doctors agreeing to the best way to treat conditions—or at least agreeing to one standard approach if evidence to support a best practice is lacking—and committing to share data and hold each other accountable in the service of consumers' getting better care. Doing what's right for patients has to be the underpinning."

The Memorial Hermann system committed to CI and invested heavily to hire practice coordinators and physician liaisons, upgrade information technology, train practices in the eClinicalWorks software, and build the infrastructure that would be the spine of CI—the clinical program committees (CPCs). This upfront investment was made based on the belief of Dan Wolterman, the system's CEO, that "if we built it [a high-quality, integrated system], they [insurers and patients] would come." Every strategy is a gamble, one that minimizes risk if well planned and thought out. Strategy is someone's best shot—without any guarantee of success—at a way to go forward.

NOTHING ATYPICAL ABOUT THE SYSTEM'S RELATIONSHIPS WITH DOCTORS

Wolterman's belief in empowering network doctors is paying off. Quality is getting better, savings are increasing, alignment is strong, and improvement is "accelerating at an accelerating pace," as network CEO Chris Lloyd has said.

But CI wasn't instantly appealing. MHMD members were initially skeptical; some saw it as an intrusion into their practice and many were concerned about the requirement to share their practice's data. Independent doctors were wary of a large and growing hospital system. Keith Fernandez, MHMD president and physician-in-chief, commented that Memorial Hermann had a traditional culture: "Nothing about the past of this system was any different from other systems—and we had a traditional hospital-centric culture. We grew as a system of hospitals, not without missteps in the eyes of some doctors."

Earlier Problems Cast Long Shadows

One worry for community-based doctors had been Memorial's acquisition of Hermann Hospital, the University of Texas (UT) Medical School's primary teaching hospital. In the late 1990s, the latter institution's survival depended on finding a financially stronger partner. When the Hermann Hospital academic doctors were folded into the newly formed Memorial Hermann system in 1997, they felt a disconnect between themselves and their suburban colleagues. In addition, community doctors distrusted the motives of executives in incorporating a teaching hospital with a troubled bottom line.

Then, in 2001, Hermann Hospital was devastated by Tropical Storm Allison. When floods took out the hospital's electrical power, five hundred patients, the Level 1 trauma service, transplant service, and speciality services were moved to other

Memorial Hermann hospitals. System CMO Michael Shabot, MD, described UT physicians' having to go to the system's community hospitals as akin to a revelation. They bonded with the community physicians and discovered that their tertiary and quaternary specialty patients could receive excellent care in community hospitals.

However, one hospital, Memorial Hermann Southwest, has been slow to shake off the baggage from an incident in 2009. The Harris County Hospital District had engaged in talks with Memorial Hermann to buy Southwest so the county could expand services to underserved populations. Two months before completing the deal, the county withdrew its offer. The plan to sell their hospital left some medical staff with a jaundiced view of administration that, until recently, has hampered their embrace of the system's improvement work at Southwest.

For their part, doctors haven't always been exemplary partners. When several doctors associated with the flagship Memorial City Hospital opted to invest in and open a facility in close proximity to it, the physicians felt that administration saw their actions as betrayal and "defection." While these doctors were running their own facility, they had stayed on the medical staff at Memorial City. That strained relationships and was symptomatic of at least some doctors' looking for more control—in that instance, ultimate control—over the inpatient setting and revenues.

Perceived Asymmetry

Three concerns imbued the physician–hospital relationship with some tension: the imbalance in power in which independent doctors felt "one down"; physicians' fears that aligning with the hospital would erode their autonomy; and lingering concerns that the system could, if it so chose, expand its employed medical group. While skepticism never escalated to bad blood, there was enough naturally occurring noise to create a slow start for alignment and CI work.

TURNING IT AROUND: DOCTORS AS FULL PARTNERS

CEO Dan Wolterman is a pragmatist; he's a politically astute leader with a deeply held commitment to doing the right thing for patients. Early on, he realized that macroeconomics would force healthcare reform and that his organization would need to change significantly to avoid collapse when payment shifted away from primarily fee-for-service. To do best by patients, the system needed to align with physicians to prepare for reforms in care delivery and reimbursement.

While Wolterman's office is on the corporate floor of an outpatient tower, he doesn't stay ensconced there; he spends a great deal of his time in the facilities. Twice a year he holds town hall meetings with the medical staff at *every one* of the system's nine hospitals. These meetings last "for as long as physicians want to stay," in Wolterman's words. What other hospital administrators might consider heretical, Wolterman sees as inevitable; and his practical viewpoint has led him to declare that the system *must* become physician-driven. Because of steps already taken to bring independent physicians closer and give them a real voice in the system, many in the MHHS organization consider him a visionary. Kimberly Rensel, a physician liaison with Memorial City Medical Center, put it this way: "He is navigating us into the future."

Leadership's authentic belief that doctors—whether employed; medical school–based; or independent, community-based—are key partners is at the core of MHMD's success. The new CI model is designed to implement physicians' hospital-related recommendations, once they're approved by hospital MECs, as well as their office-practice recommendations, once approved by MHMD's board. Shared savings are distributed to physicians when the *entire* medical staff at a hospital successfully meet targets. System governance involves MHMD physicians (who hold 5 of 25 board seats). Other physician involvement is hardwired into the network's and system's decision-making processes.

One effect of peer pressure, of an infrastructure that enables physicians to contribute in meaningful ways, of financial rewards, and of a clear compact that spells out gives and gets is that a virtuous cycle has been initiated and sustained. Physicians receive respect and responsibility, their collective performance on quality measures has earned them greater influence in the system, and, in response, their commitment to the system and clinical quality continues to deepen.

MHMD'S COMPACT: "THE WAY WE WORK"

Changing the way the system engages doctors—specifically, handing responsibility to the physician organization to develop standards for the entire system—took a leap of faith. To weather ambiguity, trusting relationships and goodwill are requisite. Chris Lloyd, CEO of MHMD, put the compact in context: "In the new world of accountable care, which, in essence, relies on population management, everyone's role has to change. Because of this, clear rules of the road were needed. As our roles as administrators have changed, the compact is the document we go to. It defines for our management how we do what we do."

Before heavy investment in CI, the physician network put nearly a year's worth of effort into creating a compact with physician members.

Creating the Compact

That effort began in 2008. At a professional meeting that year, Blakely and network CEO Scott Fenn learned of another organization's successful compact experience, led by Jack Silversin, and their interest was piqued. They sought out Silversin to learn how a compact might be useful in furthering CI. They were familiar with his involvement with Cedars-Sinai Medical Center (Los Angeles), where the medical staff had initiated a compact process in the wake of a computerized physician order entry system implementation debacle. Shabot, Cedars's chief of staff during its compact work, had been hired by Memorial Hermann as system CMO. With Shabot on board, network leadership felt there was much to be gained by having an explicit compact and were ready to commit to the process.

That retreat in early October 2008 was nearly postponed because of the devastation that Hurricane Ike dealt the Texas Gulf Coast and the city of Houston. Ike, the costliest hurricane in Texas history, came ashore on September 13. Despite the fact that the storm damaged some physicians' homes, the retreat went ahead as planned in Austin. Silversin recalls that the storm offered a more than reasonable excuse to put off the retreat, but participants wanted to go forward.

At that weekend retreat, Silversin worked with the physician network board, chiefs of staff at the hospitals, and system leaders to draft a compact between the network board and network members. Once the individuals gathered understood the concept and saw it as practical and useful, they were full speed ahead. What impressed Silversin was how quickly and deeply the group appreciated that any compact is only words on a page; the value in having agreed-on expectations is that leaders legitimately feel they have the right, and responsibility, to hold all doctors to a single standard.

The context for the weekend was how a compact could support the success of CI. The preamble drafted that weekend reads as follows:

> With Clinical Integration, HNP [former name for Memorial Hermann Health Network Providers] has introduced a new product to the Houston health care market—an interdependent network of physicians that collaborate with each other and the Memorial Hermann Hospital System to provide better-quality, highly efficient, more cost-effective care. This new product entails collective negotiation by HNP with health plans for better fees and pay-for-performance incentives.

The compact that follows identifies a reciprocal set of commitments and accountabilities between HNP's elected leaders and the physician members designed to support the organization and its members to achieve its strategic vision and build capacity to respond effectively to future challenges and opportunities.

Breaking into mixed groups, managers and physicians generated ideas for a compact. Among the elements captured from those initial discussions were the following:

- Physicians' responsibilities
  - Practice evidence-based medicine in hospital and ambulatory settings
  - Practice collaboratively with each other
  - Agree to be represented by our leaders
  - Be willing to change
  - Submit to robust peer review

- HPN board responsibilities
  - Listen
  - Provide practice management tools
  - Collate healthcare information; disseminate and use for rewards and negotiations
  - Reassure physicians that there is no direct competition from employed physicians
  - Be transparent to members

The retreat started months-long conversations about responsibilities owed by both the board and physician members for the success of CI. Discussions went on at board meetings, leadership meetings, and committee meetings. The compact development and finalization process—from the weekend retreat to a compact that defines expectations related to CI—took almost a full year. The compact that evolved details physicians' and the organization's responsibilities and is reproduced in the appendix. Exhibit 6.1 presents the attributes, as they are called, from that compact. The attributes for both "sides" were designed to be as similar as possible.

Charlotte Alexander, MD, an independent surgeon, chairs MHMD's system quality committee. She recalls the values clarification that was part of the compact development process: "Going through the compact process allowed us to clarify our values as an organization and identify what doctors wanted. A key need that surfaced was for leaders to listen and take doctors' needs into account as we move our quality and safety agenda forward. The organization has to be responsive to doctors. The compact we developed strengthens us."

Exhibit 6.1 Attributes from Memorial Hermann Physician Organization Compact

Physicians' Contributions	Board's Contributions
◆ Provide evidence-based clinical care ◆ Be transparent ◆ Collaborate ◆ Demonstrate compassion and respect ◆ Be accountable ◆ Function as a member of the MHMD team ◆ Support innovation	◆ Provide excellent governance ◆ Be transparent ◆ Collaborate ◆ Demonstrate compassion and respect ◆ Be accountable ◆ Foster a team spirit ◆ Support innovation

Source: Memorial Hermann Physician Network. Used with permission.

Living the Compact

The compact is viewed by many as an essential component of the physician network's success. It's printed on a plastic card worn by network leaders and managers. It's discussed at CPC meetings. It's a key part of the new IPA member packet. Hard copies of the compact are included in every MHMD board packet and are visible at regular "boot camp" (MHMD physician leadership development) events.

According to Shawn Griffin, MD, chief quality and informatics officer of the network, leaders' actions are guided by the principles. Griffin explains, "Compact principles have become increasingly important even if the exact language in the compact is not top-of-mind. The principles embedded in it are important as more care shifts to outpatient." Griffin reports the transformation from the earlier days of the IPA as being similar to

> going through a transition from the cruise ship metaphor to an aircraft carrier where everyone is concerned about high reliability. A lot has changed. As the compact process was starting, doctors still had reservations about MHMD being a Trojan horse—that the system would somehow take over. The success of the compact, clinical integration, and medical home all have had a lot to do with trust. The way it has worked is that doctors were granted some trust and latitude, and their work on behalf of the greater good earned them more.

The person most responsible for embedding the compact's principles into leadership's thinking and processes and for building it into CI and improvement work is Keith Fernandez, MHMD president and physician-in-chief. From all accounts,

Fernandez is the right person at the right time to help lead the transformation of the physician network. His physician peers respect him as a clinician; he still practices gastroenterology, albeit part time. He's been highly effective at keeping the compact front and center, talking about it at every CPC group meeting and every board meeting for the first two years after it was adopted. His repeated explanations of the compact's tenets helped a wide audience appreciate the reciprocity and accountability built into the document. Jon Gogola, MD, an independent obstetrician in the network, noted, "[Fernandez] is always putting this in front of CPCs saying, 'This is our compact. Remember, this is what we committed to.' Early on, specific parts of the compact were discussed at meetings; now it's the DNA of the organization." When Fernandez and Gogola meet with practices that are considering joining the network, they show them the compact. Gogola remarked, "Explaining our compact helps those on the fence understand us, and it is a way for us to be more comfortable in discussing our mission and how we work."

Using the compact—in meaningful ways—is what makes it so potent at MHMD. Fernandez reflects on walking the walk:

> Here's one example of its impact on my leadership. Physicians will call me when they're frustrated because something has gone wrong in their eyes. Given the spirit of the compact, I need to look at the situation from their point of view. I need to hear and understand their side of the story, not dismiss or minimize it. As a doctor myself—one representing the organization—I look at the compact and it leads me to having a different conversation—which always works. My common response is to say, "Let me understand your view and I'll be your advocate."

In 2012, the network overstepped, in some physicians' eyes, by sending a letter to patients under physicians' names without first clearing it with network members. When the ire surfaced, Fernandez reached out to all who were affected, even those who had not complained, calling them to apologize and taking some to dinner. Offering no excuses, he took full responsibility. As a result of his recovery efforts, some of the affected doctors "are among our most loyal advocates now," according to Fernandez.

CLINICAL INTEGRATION: IT WORKS

Today's successful CI—based on network physicians' participation on CPCs to generate system-wide policy—is inextricably linked to the MHMD compact.

How It Functions

In 2010 there were 18 CPCs; today there are 47. According to Leticia Mireles, director of clinical programs at MHMD, they are flourishing. A typical CPC has 2 physician members from each of the system's hospitals. To populate committees, Mireles solicits recommendations from hospital CEOs, CMOs, and MHMD board members. The physician CPC member must be one of the 2,000 physicians who are officially sanctioned as "clinically integrated" (agreeing to meet requirements for transparency, data sharing, using MHMD clinical software, and being eligible for savings distributions). Mireles explained, "Physicians are dying to be on the committees. I get calls all the time asking how I can get on a CPC." The percentage of clinically integrated network members who have sat on a committee is significant. With about 20 doctors on each of 40 committees, and 5 to 30 physicians on 17 task forces, that means about half of the 2,000 have played, or are currently playing, an active role. The phenomenon of "like attracting like" is becoming more evident and helpful to the process.

CPCs usually meet on weeknights. For attending meetings, committee members are paid a modest stipend that acknowledges their effort and contributions; most have family, personal, or other commitments competing for off-hours time. Mireles, with a staff of two, supports the committees' work and helps chairs set agendas. For new committees, Fernandez sets the context and describes the need for the work the group is about to undertake. A CPC might meet only two or three times to formulate a new policy or suggest a change, or it might meet for several months.

The beauty of the program is that physicians themselves hash out their differences to come up with recommendations. Mireles reports that in committee meetings, transparency trumps protection: "The place most of our physicians on committees have gotten to is, 'We need to put up our data—how else can we improve?'" Committees are multidisciplinary. Each has 20 or so physicians; nursing, pharmacy, and, often, case management are represented (as voting members). Following formal adoption and implementation of a committee's recommendations, the question in hospitals or among practices is, Why not follow protocols your doctor peers generated on your behalf? At MHMD, you won't hear, Administration is making us do this, and what do they know about quality anyway?

In addressing controversy, the CPCs have consistently done the right thing—at MHMD, defined as "doing what's best for the patient." One CPC addressed neurosurgeons' use of multiple vendors in the hospitals. There had been 7 vendors of spinal implants. For the 9 CEOs of hospitals where neurosurgery is performed, a conversation to limit choice would have been difficult at best. But the neurosurgery

CPC included 18 neurosurgeons who met over a few months and narrowed the number of vendors to 2. This decision, adopted systemwide, saved millions of dollars and was handled from start to finish by clinicians, not administrators. In the past five years, CPCs have passed numerous recommendations, including capped pricing on orthopedic vendors used systemwide and a guideline requiring ultrasound for central-line insertion. A CPC also standardized peer-review procedures and a scoring form used across the system. Another time, the orthopedic CPC turned down a high-volume surgeon's request for 2 new pieces of equipment. The committee ruled that the orthopedic surgeon would need to provide evidence that the equipment would improve care and lower cost.

The CPC decisions also affect safety and hospital spending. One approved recommendation requires every patient admitted to be weighed; approximating or accepting the patient's word is no longer accepted because accurate weight is essential for drug dosing. That recommendation obliges administration to buy many more scales. The system's obligation is to find the resources to do so after a well-thought-out and debated measure is passed.

Joint operating committees (JOCs) address cross-departmental quality issues that fall within the purview of two or more CPC committees. A JOC was convened to recommend a standard for deep vein thrombosis prophylaxis that used the pulmonary specialty association guidelines as a starting point; it worked with representatives from many specialty committees to generate a MHMD standard. Management of bariatric patients in the emergency department was a cross-specialty JOC initiative.

Every two months, a full CPC meeting convenes the chairs from all CPCs. In the fall of 2013, the full CPC heard reports from 22 committees—together, they made 57 recommendations.

"Up and Over"

Coined by system CMO Shabot, "up and over" refers to the mechanism by which the CPCs' quality and safety guidelines get approved and implemented in hospitals. Recommendations approved by the full CPC go "up" to the MHMD board and then the system board's quality committee (SQC). If approved there, they go "over" to each hospital's chief of staff and CEO for consideration by their MEC. As one executive said, this structure sends the message to CPCs: "You tell us what to do and we'll do it." At each hospital, the SQC-approved recommendations go before the MEC for a straight up-or-down vote to adopt the measure. When an MEC votes to not accept a measure, the chief of staff and CEO of that hospital are asked to attend the next SQC meeting to explain their rationale for rejecting a physician-originated measure. In one instance, the critical care CPC had approved the requirement for ultrasound guidance for central-line insertion; this requirement was initially accepted by only six of nine MECs (in the relevant hospitals). It took nearly a year for all nine to sign off on it.

Delegating this level of authority to doctors has served several key purposes for MHHS. There is a smoothly operating procedure for the system hospitals to jointly develop and adopt order sets, policies, and protocols. Because that work is done "by doctors for doctors," hospital CEOs are relieved of having to deny or grant individual physicians' requests—thus, to a large degree, taking management out of the "bad guy" role. By giving important work to physicians, it binds them to the system's quality agenda; moreover, when physicians follow the guidelines, quality improves and they benefit financially. Most important, it helps restore physicians' professional decision-making authority, which has been progressively diminished by payers, regulators, and other forces. Last, it has a positive impact on relationships. Griffin notes, "Progress on both quality and trust among doctors and between doctors and administration has been accelerating. Doctors have shown they can be trusted, and we have shown the system can be trusted."

Recognition and Peer Pressure Support MHMD's Quality Agenda

At the start of 2013, Fernandez wanted to recognize the effort CPC participants have put into their work. He set aside funds for an award program. He asked CPC committee chairs to rank the work of all CPCs over the past 12 months; the top five would each receive a cash award that they could spend for quality and safety. Votes were tallied and winning CPCs recognized, but after nearly a year only one committee had requested and used its allotted award (for clinical research). The recognition by peers did have great meaning and ultimately was all that was needed. It is striking how effectively the CPCs and the overall CI strategy at Memorial Hermann have leveraged nonmonetary recognition (trust and respect earning greater influence in decisions), physicians' innate competitiveness, peer pressure—and the desire to be inside the "inner ring."[2]

There is no clear evidence that, in building their CI program, MHMD leaders consciously took advantage of the inner-ring dynamic—that is, the dynamic that drives people's desire to join exclusive clubs. However, one can't help but be struck by the virtuous cycle now operating at MHMD and the growing credibility, influence, professional satisfaction, and financial reward that accrue to those physicians who own the system vision and are aligned with it. An inner ring is establishing itself. When asked what they felt accounted for the success of the CI work, physicians interviewed at MHMD most commonly responded that quality-oriented physicians want to associate with like-minded others.

If all the medical staff in a hospital meet CPC-established targets, then those who are clinically integrated are eligible for a bonus (the distribution of which is also decided by a committee of doctors). However, their interest in getting "in the game" can't be chalked up to a few thousand dollars at the end of the year. Financial incentives have some role, but they also carry the risk of extinguishing internal motivation (Frey and Osterloh 2012; Kohn 1993; Pink 2009).

The Inner-Ring Role of the Compact

In supporting the success of CI, the MHMD compact plays a significant role. It specifies the running rails of the relationship between the network and its physician members. But it also explicitly states what it takes to be "in"; that is, what an independent, contracted, or employed doctor has to do to gain admission to the clinically integrated inner ring.

Because the program is set up for *some* to be financially rewarded only if *all* medical staff meet the standard peers have set, the motivation to help "all boats rise" is built in. Because a weak link has implications for the entire chain, the compact's expectations have been cited to help move physicians out of the CI program who could not or would not follow physician-generated guidelines. While this might sound punitive, those in the network don't see it that way. They are engaged with their hospital system in a win for patients, for the system, and for themselves.

The bonus alone cannot account for the push for quality at MHMD; the motivation for living the compact goes well beyond tangible rewards. Gogola believes that abiding by it helps secure his preferred future: "Our values are embedded in our compact, and these came out of a lot of discussion. Basically, shouldn't we expect these of ourselves? Our independence is maintained by participating in the network and following the compact."

A Long Journey

System CEO Wolterman believes employing doctors takes away their entrepreneurial edge. His conviction is that the best model for a care delivery system is one that builds on independent physicians. He said, "We set out to show we can get similar outcomes to those of fully employed medical groups like Geisinger and Mayo.

No other organization had been able to match their results. I also knew when we started that getting cooperation and bringing 3,900 independent doctors into a high-functioning, high-quality IPA would be a Herculean task."

He returned again and again to his belief that fee-for-service was unsustainable and that the market would shift away from it. Until recently, when doctors dedicated time to improvement and got better outcomes, the savings would accrue to the hospital—the market wasn't rewarding doctors yet for quality. Wolterman describes the struggle to maintain the CI model as follows: "This was not a straight line to success but a journey with a lot of pitfalls. In the mid-2000s some of my executive team felt it was time to pull the plug, but I said, 'No, I believe we need a fully integrated physician network.' It took faith to keep it going and we are fortunate things did move in our direction."

Reflecting on the value of the compact, he comments, "The compact gave 3,900 independent physicians a common behavioral platform. Having that platform is critical—without it, there is divergent behavior leading to miscommunication and doctor-to-doctor issues. The compact helps calm that down by laying down principles for how to communicate and behave. It allowed us to move expeditiously toward the goal of becoming an integrated system."

A SYSTEM THAT THRIVES THROUGH SHARED POWER

The system board has five members who are independent physicians. When that board was streamlined a couple of years ago, in response to Dan Wolterman's recommendation, the system board created the Physicians Council to be an advisory group to the board.

The Physicians Council meets in executive session with the system board without executives present, demonstrating the trust the system has placed in its physicians. Twenty-four physicians sit on the council. In addition, as we've seen, the structure through which CPCs' recommendations reach the system board's quality committee is populated with physicians. These hardwired opportunities for input and influence affirm the value that MHHS places on engaging physicians (Exhibit 6.2).

"Medical group without walls" is a term that's been around for a long time. The Memorial Hermann physician network is at a point where the phrase aptly applies to its two thousand clinically integrated physicians. With its compact work, success with CI, the availability of shared savings, and truly valuing physicians, Memorial Hermann Health System is able to get ahead of and prepare for the reform wave that is likely to pummel others without such committed physicians.

Exhibit 6.2 Structures That Hardwire Physician Influence into MHHS Decision Making

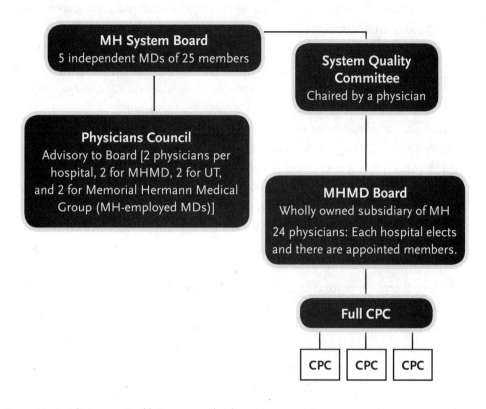

Source: Memorial Hermann Health System. Used with permission.

SUMMING UP

Chuck Stokes, system COO: "This healthcare system is becoming more physician driven. At the end of the day, it's physicians who control cost and quality. Nothing happens in the hospital until the physician decides to admit a patient—nothing happens unless the physician prescribes or orders it. Therefore, the engagement of doctors and their trust is key to our success."

This success isn't the result of any single action. It does, however, represent the confluence of several factors:

1. Leaders, in conjunction with front-line physicians, developed programs that resonate with physicians.
   - The rationale for CI and standards for care is couched in language that speaks to clinicians: This is about patient care.

- Transparency around data, discussions at regional meetings, and the sharing of unblinded results all tap into the way physicians were trained and like to learn.
- Independence is highly valued: The network has found a way to support important aspects of autonomy (being your own business). The trade-off is that one must commit to follow the compact; and for the two thousand core, clinically integrated doctors, it's a win-win.

2. CEO Wolterman put forward a vision of the future that makes sense to physicians and that positions the whole system to be ahead of the curve. He speaks of MHHS's becoming "physician driven." His ceding some control to the doctors is cited as pivotal. He appreciates that physician engagement is the critical ingredient in care coordination and is willing to let go of the reins as physicians step up and work for the system's success. He is credible when talking about the future and he maintains a visible presence in the nine hospitals.

3. A high degree of mutual trust and respect exists between leaders of the network and physician members. Fernandez is lauded as an effective physician leader, eloquent speaker, and person of high integrity. The doctors believe he has their backs. His words and actions set the tone for respectful relationships.

4. Virtuous cycles operate that lead the quality agenda to "accelerate at an accelerating pace."
- System leaders put responsibility for system-wide recommendations into the hands of independent doctors. In actively improving quality, safety, and efficiency, these doctors have earned more respect and five seats at the system board table. In addition, the Physicians Council was created to advise the board. Trust and respect produced results that engendered more (mutual) trust and respect, and real influence for independent physicians.
- Fernandez's insistence that CPCs put patients' interests first and foremost sets the tone for committee discussions. Although doing the right thing for patients turns out to produce economic gains for doctors—reinforcement for keeping the focus on clinical quality and safety—patient care, not money, is the motivation behind CPC recommendations.

5. Peer pressure and like-mindedness both play key roles.
- The bulk of physicians in the CI program are like-minded. The phenomenon "like seeks like" plays a significant role in shifting the overall mindset toward patient-centeredness. The more those who share a

patient-centered orientation coalesce, the more the "inner ring" phenomenon takes hold. Because they are by nature competitive, more
doctors want "in."

- ◆ Recommendations for policies, protocols, and other decisions are created by doctors for doctors (nurses also have a vote). While local hospital administration has to ensure that any physician *mis*behavior that may
  occur is effectively dealt with by medical staff peer-review mechanisms,
  for the most part they are not the "heavies" trying to force physicians
  to change their practices. Within the CPCs, peers hash out views and
  arrive at a recommendation; then they talk with other doctors at their
  hospitals. When a doctor's performance is below standard in a regional
  group, another doctor offers help. Doctors take it upon themselves to
  have potentially difficult peer-to-peer conversations; they don't lateral
  most issues to network administrators.
- ◆ The group nature of the incentives means that every doctor has a vested
  interest in all doctors' doing well. Beyond getting better managed-care
  contracts, individuals earn bonuses (distribution decided by fellow doctors) for meeting quality measures *as a group*. The amount is not insig-
  nificant; as one put it, "It's not enough to buy a car, but it's an awfully
  nice vacation."

6. Leaders genuinely appreciate that the elixir for partnering with independent
   doctors to improve care is building and sustaining respectful relationships.
   Toward that end, the compact spells out the rules of engagement, and network leaders make conscious efforts to live up to their commitments. The
   compact has real meaning through

   - ◆ decision making by the MHMD board;
   - ◆ selecting practices most likely to fit with the developing network ethos;
   - ◆ onboarding and separating out practices that demonstrate little willing-
     ness to "join the club"; and
   - ◆ executives' talking about it—giving it visibility and importance.

NOTES

1. Memorial Hermann Health System's and MHMD's awards include The
   Joint Commission and National Quality Forum (NQF) John M. Eisenberg
   Award for Patient Safety and Quality; the Truven Health Top 5 Large
   Health Systems Award; the NQF National Quality Healthcare Award;
   and the National Health System Patient Safety Leadership Award (given

jointly by VHA Foundation and National Business Group on Health). Healthgrades rated 4 of the system's hospitals among America's 50 best; and the system was a finalist for the AHA-McKesson Quest for Quality prize. In 2011, the care management division was awarded the Franklin Award of Distinction by The Joint Commission and the American Care Management Association.

2. In a lecture he delivered in 1944, the English novelist and moralist C. S. Lewis noted the strong pull that the desire to be part of the "in crowd" has on most people, though he didn't define "in." Lewis applied the term "inner ring" to the ubiquitous cliques and closed societies, large and small, that those on the outside perceive as exclusive and therefore want to be part of. To quote Lewis, "I believe that in all men's lives at certain periods, and in many men's lives at all periods between infancy and extreme old age, one of the most dominant elements is the desire to be inside the local Ring and the terror of being left outside."

    Pulitzer Prize winner Tina Rosenberg (2011) has written extensively about what she calls "the social cure," or the potent role peer pressure plays in any number of change programs or interventions. Her 2011 best-selling book, *Join the Club: How Peer Pressure Can Change the World,* provides multiple examples of persuading people to make choices they would rather avoid—not by information or education campaigns, but by tapping into a deep-seated human need "to belong, to be part of the in crowd, to be loved, admired and respected. These programs change personal behavior through social pressure." The medical profession is itself an exclusive club, one that is joined only via rigorous training, has its own code of conduct (Hippocratic oath), and has outward symbols of privilege (short, and then long white coats).

CHAPTER 7

Salem Hospital: Management and Medical Staff Heal a Fractured Relationship at a Community Hospital

All routes out of our problems in health care—the big ones at least—traverse the meadows of cooperation.
—*Don Berwick, MD*

Don Berwick penned those words in 2000 for the foreword to the first edition of the book I co-wrote with Jack Silversin, *Leading Physicians Through Change: How to Achieve and Sustain Results*. Berwick drew this conclusion from observing how mistrust, thinly veiled resentments, and lack of civility impede the work healthcare organizations carry out—treating, healing, and comforting patients and families. Simply put, we, and Berwick, have repeatedly witnessed unhealthy and unconstructive relationships present significant barriers to delivering on the promise of better, safer, more efficient care. There is no way around this truth; all successful improvement work and care coordination necessitate strong working relationships.

Salem Hospital is the sole acute-care hospital in Salem, Oregon. Salem is located in the Willamette Valley, known for its prize-winning Pinot Noir wines. Wine enthusiasts talk of "terroir" as the site-specific climate, soil, and weather conditions that affect the unique characteristics of a wine. In the case of this hospital and its medical staff, one aspect of the terroir affecting their relationship is the fact that Salem Hospital is the only hospital in town. Another anomaly is the degree to which physicians in Salem are still largely independent; in other parts of the state, doctors are becoming employed in significant numbers.

Salem Hospital's experience illustrates how developing a compact can start to heal a deep rift between doctors and administrators who harbored not just suspicions but hostility toward one other. Their compact work offers a view into how troubled or contentious relationships can be put on a better footing through dialogue and keeping commitments.

TENSIONS ESCALATE

It is not uncommon to find some tension between administrators and physicians—that is, between the people responsible for budgeting, operations, and strategy and those who deliver patient care. As discussed in Chapter 1, their work differs significantly, as do their professional training and scope of responsibility. At Salem, these inherent tensions had spiraled to a level that could have jeopardized new initiatives.

A critical impetus for Salem's decision to undertake compact work was that a significant number of community physicians viewed almost every management action as suspicious. Anything less than total transparency was deemed intentional withholding of information. A history of mistrust, accusations of dishonest motives, and local doctors' legislative action against the hospital were taking a toll on everyone. The pool of goodwill that must exist in a successful organization was almost empty; Salem faced a parched landscape with little leeway for missteps. No one was cutting anyone else any slack.

When the Past Isn't Past

When any relationship sours, usually a multitude of things are going wrong—and that holds true for the hospital–doctor relationship in Salem. In 1969, two hospitals merged to create Salem Hospital, making it, as noted, the only acute-care hospital in the city. Some people, including Cort Garrison, MD, the hospital's chief information officer, point to the hospital's monopolistic position as the foundation of the strife. "People need choice—and for the physicians in this community, there is no choice," Garrison said. More important than loss of perceived bargaining power is physicians' knowing that they cannot leverage that power whether they wish to or not. Garrison speaks from experience. He is a practicing physician in the community and had held a number of positions as a member of the medical staff—including vice president and then president—before taking up his administrative position.

For its part, the hospital wasn't helpful in dispelling physicians' perceptions that they were "one down" in this relationship. Years before, physicians had proposed joint venturing with the hospital to open several surgi-centers, but the administration stepped away because it would not have total control. (Legally, as a nonprofit entity, the hospital arguably needed full responsibility but did not do an adequate job communicating this issue to physicians.) The doctors went ahead independently and still operate several freestanding outpatient centers. The way that the deal unfolded reinforced opinions that the hospital wasn't interested in a true partnership with local physicians.

For whatever reasons—the personality of former executives and the physicians' actions might each have played a role—administrators defaulted to a mind-set of suspicion toward physicians' commitment to the institution. A gap in trust and understanding led both parties to interpret well-intentioned decisions through a negative lens. A culture developed in which it was standard operating procedure for administrators to make decisions affecting medical staff without involving staff. (Physicians' actions undoubtedly played some role in this unilateral decision-making.) From the administrators' perspective, they and the board always had in mind the best interests of the community; that was their responsibility.

Executive Leadership Issues

Before Norm Gruber became CEO, the hospital's executive leadership had been homegrown, rising through the ranks to the C-suite. This practice was common in the past. The naïveté of the former CEO was evident in a decision he made that reverberated through the medical community for more than ten years.

In 2000, Oregon developed a strategy to upgrade trauma response statewide. Representatives visited every hospital in the state, including Salem, to encourage proposals for the hospitals to become certified as Level II trauma centers. The Salem Hospital medical staff and board were not included in these conversations, and when doctors read in the newspaper about the proposal the CEO had developed, they pushed back hard, causing the plan to be dropped. The CEO had begun the certification process without malice but also without appreciating the implications it could have for doctors' practice lives. A significant rift in trust resulted.

Salem Hospital trustees are not unlike trustees who serve on local hospital boards across the country: Nonphysician members tend to be civic-oriented business people or leaders of organizations other than hospitals. They volunteer time and effort to help ensure the viability of an important, and often cherished, community asset. A patient-oriented, financially healthy hospital that scores high on quality helps attract talent to local businesses and positively contributes to the community's well-being. A business executive who, in his or her own organization, communicates the importance of a policy and sees it take effect in short order, is flummoxed that the hospital seems to operate in a different reality. That person's view may be: "Just tell the doctors what we need to get done. Period. Full stop." Especially when the potential for patient harm is real, many trustees don't have patience for or understanding of the intricacies and traditions that make meaningful and sustained change a challenge.

In Salem, a lack of sensitivity—going both ways—contributed to the widening breach of trust. One board member who felt an urgent need for faster improvement shared her concerns at a general medical staff meeting. But the doctors present heard her concerns as a dressing down; they felt disrespected. The data about safety incidents that had lit a fire under the board hadn't been shared with the doctors. There was a disconnect in understanding the situation and who needed to do what. This incident, considered by many at the hospital to be the nadir of a tense relationship, left many feeling deeply troubled.

CHALLENGES IN MOVING BEYOND "GOOD ENOUGH"

Since 1898, Salem Hospital has had only ten CEOs. Long tenures and promoting from within had led to insular views. Prior to the late 1990s, the hospital board was similarly made up of long-serving leaders. Board members had term limits but selected their replacements; so, for the most part, the board carried on, decade to decade, with like-minded individuals. The board's view for some time had been that the hospital was "good enough" for Salem. Not seeing any competitors on the horizon, the board felt no need to push boundaries or focus on being more patient-centric. It was assumed local patients would always fill the beds.

A New Board, a New CEO: A New Vision

In the late 1990s, board membership changed and a new mind-set took hold. Members became active proponents of a new vision for the hospital and wanted someone to lead it in a different way to bring the hospital into the twenty-first century. In 2003, the board selected Norm Gruber—the hospital's first out-of-house and professional CEO—to spearhead a transformation. One qualification that made Gruber an attractive candidate was his prior experience in San Diego, a market much more competitive than Salem. Gruber's mandate from the board included changing the culture to be in sync with the vision of a safe, high-quality, patient-centered institution.

A Chief Medical Officer Who Relates to Physicians
Gruber took that charge in hand. In 2005, he hired David Holloway as chief medical officer (CMO). Holloway, who has since left his position at Salem Hospital, was well versed in quality and safety improvement and had a history of building relationships with physicians. His previous work experience included collegial

relationships between doctors and administration, and constructive interactions in a system where he led physician integration. Immediately prior to his post at Salem Hospital, Holloway was part of the executive team in a hospital system that experienced tension because doctors could leave one hospital for another if their needs were not met. However, none of that experience had prepared him for the state of the doctor–hospital relationship in Salem, where, in his words, "What I found was a situation where there was plenty of room for improvement—on both sides."

A Patient-Oriented Building Program
In line with the board's vision for Salem Hospital, an ambitious building program was undertaken. Gruber secured funding for significant renovation to the campus, including a new building housing a modern emergency department, operating rooms, imaging, a catheterization lab, and 120 inpatient beds; a new central energy plant; a regional laboratory; and a new outpatient rehabilitation building. Nursing units were refreshed. All new facilities and upgrades were guided by evidence-based design to create physical spaces that help patients recover in a safer environment and help make staff jobs easier. Attempts to unfreeze some aspects of the former culture and begin anew went hand in hand with the physical transformation of the campus; both the culture and the building program were aimed at "upping the game" and creating a modern, patient-centered institution.

The physicians had mixed reactions to these changes. Some doctors shared the leadership's vision for the future, and the medical executive committee wanted to do the right thing. Pockets of doctors actively engaged in work to improve quality, believing that, with doctor involvement, the hospital could be second to none. But the transformation did not energize all physicians; many felt that the changes Gruber had instigated were not part of the deal they had signed up for as members of the medical staff.

Skepticism of Administration's Motives

A significant number of medical staff members didn't understand the need for change. Leadership of the local physician organization—to which almost all community-based doctors belong—held (and, to some extent, still holds) a cynical view of Gruber's motives. Some saw a threat in the hospital's employing physicians, believing that Gruber would prefer to employ *all* the hospital's physicians, without concern for the livelihood of long-standing members of the medical community. Some simply did not like Gruber's style; plain-speaking and direct, he did not sugarcoat the message that doctors needed to change. Physicians have excellent memories. In the early days of Gruber's tenure, a few vice presidents had demonstrated an our-way-or-the-highway attitude. Even though they were moved out, resentment toward administration simmered. Some in the community still hold grudges that predate Gruber's arrival.

Inadequate Physician Accountability

When Gruber arrived, he felt there had been too little physician accountability. The peer-review process did not deal with behavioral issues and disrespect; it tolerated some egregious behaviors. A high priority for Gruber was to develop a culture where the members of the medical staff take responsibility for peers' behavior. He pushed to make physicians more accountable.

Lifting the rock labeled "reluctance to review peers," one finds unexamined expectations held in common by physicians. Physicians' proclivity to give each other wide latitude and their discomfort in giving colleagues constructive feedback are symptomatic of a psychological contract built on personal autonomy, entitlement, and protection. Central to this compact are the shared beliefs that "there but for the grace of God go I; mistakes happen; negatively reviewing a peer leaves me vulnerable to others' critique." The unwritten compact among many Salem-area physicians held that the hospital was the workshop where they practiced medicine. They delivered good care as they defined it, admitted patients, served on committees, participated in the occasional town hall meeting, met continuing medical education requirements, and fulfilled their professional obligations as best they could. That's the deal they signed onto. The call to hold each other more accountable—from someone who was not a physician—threatened the old compact and, without being framed as such, was perceived as an attack on professionalism.

Employing Physicians Exacerbates Tension

Many hospitals are challenged to maintain positive relationships with community-based physicians while building an employed group. When competition is involved and physician livelihoods are at stake, there are few easy answers. To both compete and cooperate takes a mature relationship, one in which all parties can discuss their shared interests (i.e., an economically viable hospital and the ability to attract physician talent) and acknowledge competing needs. Sometimes the best outcome is that parties agree to disagree—and not blow their relationship to smithereens—knowing, at the end of the day, that they are interdependent.

As Salem Hospital built an employed group over the past decade, economic issues became another threat to the hospital–physician relationship. There was little controversy over the hiring of psychiatrists or trauma surgeons, but the hospital's employment of primary care physicians became a third-rail issue. The hospital identified a need for more primary care capacity than local doctors were willing to supply; of concern was a critical shortage of practices to take on Medicare patients. Even though proactive conversations had made the case for employing primary care doctors, most doctors felt that, in principle, the hospital should not create competition. By all accounts, the hospital's primary care group got off to a rough start. Attracted by commitments that the practice would be set up as a medical home and that registries would be created to help manage chronic-disease patients, some doctors left within a couple of years because promised supports did not materialize as quickly as expected.

After some early turnover, Willamette Health Partners is now a 100-provider group that includes physicians (doctors of medicine and doctors of osteopathy) and nurse practitioners, 11 of whom are primary care. Much of the heat around this issue has dissipated because most employed physicians are specialists or are not able to provide services to the community, based on reimbursement, without the hospital's subsidization. However, some doctors are still wary of the hospital's move to employ physicians and, for them, it remains a troublesome issue.

Adaptive Changes Are Hard to Accept and Risky to Lead

Finally, many Salem physicians were unprepared for the adaptive nature of the changes that leadership had set in motion. Disappointment and anger are not unusual when a new regime takes action to improve matters. Ronald Heifetz and Marty Linsky (2002a, 31), in *Leadership on the Line: Staying Alive Through the Dangers of Leading*, spell out the ways that disaffected members of an organization strike out at leaders who upend the status quo: "When exercising leadership, you risk getting marginalized, diverted, attacked or seduced. Regardless of the form, however, the point is the same. When people resist adaptive work, their goal is to shut down those who exercise leadership in order to preserve what they have." Too much change too fast—with inadequate attention to the adjustments in routines, patterns, beliefs, and even values of those asked to change—is certain to generate pushback.

WHAT HAPPENED IN SALEM CAN HAPPEN ANYWHERE

Salem Hospital's situation reflects a perfect storm of actions and reactions that can be found, perhaps in less destructive combinations, in almost any community hospital. When a dysfunctional relationship affects organizational performance or business success, the point has been reached where it doesn't matter which party bears most responsibility. In this community, both doctors and administration were seeing each other solely through their own lenses, which had become shaded and fixed. In their seminal work on negotiation, *Getting Together*, Roger Fisher and Scott Brown (1988, 25) observed, "Each of us tends to see things in ways that take our own interests disproportionately into account. And the facts we know best are those closest to us."

Building a positive relationship would mean finding a means to unfreeze views, look anew at some facts, and learn to relate in new ways. In then-CMO Holloway's words, "The compact creates a containment vessel for having really difficult conversations without it blowing up."

BUILDING COMMON GROUND

Salem Hospital's tripartite compact reflects the board's active involvement in its development. It also reflects initiatives, predating that work, to educate the board and foster partnership with both administration and medical staff for quality improvement.

Realization That a Shared Vision Is Needed

Within months of starting as CMO, Holloway introduced the Institute of Healthcare Improvement (IHI) "Boards on Board" initiative, an educational campaign to inform board members of how they can be active participants in improving care. Although boards may consider this work to be solely the business of the medical executive committee, because reimbursement is increasingly linked to quality, all boards need to be concerned with this issue. Oregon statutes hold trustees ultimately responsible for the quality of medical care delivered.

In 2010, Holloway generated a broader conversation about the extent to which doctors and board members had shared goals. He posed two questions: Does the majority of the medical staff understand the direction of the board of trustees? Does the board of trustees understand the direction of the medical staff? Discussions at the board level and with groups of doctors pointed out the need for a vision for which *all* stakeholders felt ownership. "Common ground" became associated with work on the shared vision, and the phrase was attached to the ensuing compact process.

Decision to Take on Compact Work

Holloway heard Jack Silversin talk about compacts in an IHI Annual Forum workshop in 2003. He was already familiar with our model that posits shared vision, effective physician leadership, and an explicit compact—aligned with the vision—as critical in forming a foundation for successful change efforts (Kornacki and Silversin 2012, 9). Holloway brought the message to Salem that all three components—not a compact in isolation—would need attention if the organization was to build change capacity. He continued to attend IHI conferences with Salem colleagues so they could discuss lessons that could be applied back home. Among those joining Holloway at a 2008 IHI event was Alan Costic, current board chair at Salem Hospital. Costic had been on the board for a couple of years and had concerns over the state of the hospital–doctor relationship. CEO Gruber's exploration of Lean took him to several organizations—including Virginia Mason Medical Center, where he learned about the connection between that organization's approach to Lean and its physician compact.

Holloway championed the compact work while moving the organization forward on the need for a shared vision and building physician leadership. He hoped these discussions, especially around the compact, would foster more productive relationships. "Too often," he told me, "I see individuals reflexively run up the ladder of inference and make quick assumptions that only inflame the situation." Holloway reasoned that if hospital administrators and medical staff got it right, their compact process would allow for healthy dialogue that included nonjudgmental inquiry of others' perspectives, balanced with advocacy of individuals' interests. He was not interested in a process that drove through to a final document without the rich conversation that would allow all to feel heard and to draw a line under the past.

An expanding group understood the usefulness of an explicit physician compact, through reading about it or attending Silversin's workshops. A small cluster—the joint conference committee (JCC), which included the board chair and vice chair; the medical staff president and president-elect; Holloway; and Gruber—formed to sort out different perspectives on quality of care. From their conversations, they recognized the need for some common vision and invited Silversin to share the idea of a compact. In the spring of 2011, Silversin spoke at a series of town hall meetings, held throughout one day, to expose more of the medical staff to this concept and to build support for doing this work. Holloway commented, "Even though I and others felt we should try to create a compact, it couldn't be my call alone. Through the town halls, we attempted to bring medical staff into a conversation about the value and timing of our taking this on." Participant feedback was given to the JCC, which decided the response was positive enough to go forward. This marked an important transition in the process: recognition by a number of people that it was important to heal the medical staff–administration relationship.

Four doctors were added to the JCC to form the Common Ground steering committee, designated as the group that would guide the compact process. This group identified the following goals:

- Build a community of physicians and hospital leaders whose behavior demonstrates a deep appreciation that they are interdependent for success.
- Develop a written, final shared vision statement and compact with wide input and buy-in.
- Increase capacity to provide and receive constructive feedback and support for improvement.

THE NUTS AND BOLTS OF THE PROCESS

Defining a Shared Vision

In the late summer of 2011, the Common Ground process got under way with a retreat to define a shared vision for the organization's future. That fall, the steering committee held multiple meetings via video link with Silversin to refine the language for a vision that would be the foundation for any compact; to deepen members' understanding of what new expectations could mean; and to help members get to know each other, clear the air, and build trust. This phase was not rushed: Getting deep buy-in among those on the steering committee was key to this process. In most compacts I've been involved with, physicians are asked to put autonomy in perspective and be open to evidence-based medicine. Those are significant adjustments. Add in the suspicions that hung over administration's motives, and this compact process could have been seen as "consultant speak" or as a management manifesto.

To be effective sponsors, this key steering group needed to coalesce. In the beginning, participants were tense and skeptical. With Silversin facilitating the discussions via video conferencing, the group began to open up and even aired dirty laundry. A pivotal moment occurred when a doctor aired his views on the hospital's hiring of doctors who would compete with independent ones. Trustee Bonnie Driggers responded, "I've never heard it like this before." Her acknowledgment that she understood that decision's ramifications in a totally different way broke down some reserve. She demonstrated how listening and not being defensive opens up possibilities. This breakthrough helped the group develop trust and what was to become a strong commitment to the effort. Holloway reflected that much of the progress the steering committee made through the fall and winter was the result of not letting elephants sit in the room unaddressed.

Next Steps

Expanding the Leadership

The steering committee formed a guiding coalition of individuals who were seen to have legitimate authority (elected by medical staff) and physicians who had demonstrated an interest in leadership. This coalition was composed of the medical executive committee, section chiefs, and doctors and managers who had attended the first round of leadership development offered under the auspices of the hospital's Physician Leadership Institute (PLI). All participated in a workshop with Silversin to prepare them (1) to be able advocates for the compact in informal discussions and (2) to play constructive roles during medical staff section meetings to vet the compact. This guiding coalition was invited to the subsequent two retreats that hammered out the draft compact and the final version after feedback had been collected.

Drafting the Compact

In spring 2012, a second retreat resulted in the draft compact. The mixing of trustees, managers, and physicians stood out as "not business as usual." Participants came with entirely different attitudes than in the past—neither blaming nor dismissive. The quality of conversation and appreciation for others' views became the hallmarks of that retreat and the subsequent one. Conversation—even down to framing the document's wording—was candid and, at times, edgy. Participants had strong feelings about the meaning of words and they did not hold back their feelings. It felt as though a new chapter was opening and that it was possible for all stakeholders to be on the same page.

Getting Broad Input

Then–board chair Ken Sherman knew that the next challenge would be expanding the number of those able to converse constructively and support the compact. He likened this challenge to being asked by a friend to describe a movie you just saw:

"It's not possible to convey the actual experience. You can talk about the plot line, but you need to see the movie for yourself to appreciate it and get its meaning. Words aren't sufficient; only first-hand experience would help others really understand the compact."

With a draft in hand, the steering committee was ready to meet with small groups of medical staff to solicit reactions and input to the shared vision and compact. Nearly 30 medical staff section meetings were held that fall. CMO Holloway, along with a board member and a physician from the steering committee, discussed the compact, which people had in advance, and solicited reactions. Compact discussions also took place in quarterly staff meetings and in departments. Gruber reported, "Wordsmithing that happened at meetings where the compact was discussed was not unimportant. We needed to come to a shared meaning of what key words or concepts really mean. What 'communication' or 'accountability' mean to a manager might be different from what a doctor means by those words. The very process of creating the compact and having dialogue about what words or phrases mean is as important as the final document."

The compact (reproduced in full in the appendix) evolved as feedback was collected and medical staff had an opportunity to participate in a final review session. The compact was considered final and approved at the third retreat meeting, held in November 2012. The organization produced a compact brochure that presents the board's responsibilities, the hospital's, and medical staff's. The brochure's illustrations convey the idea of shared and unique commitments and serve as an example of the power of graphics. Exhibit 7.1 highlights one tenet from each of the four parts of the full document.

Implementation: The CIC

At that third retreat, the steering group chartered the compact implementation committee (CIC) to explore how to embed the compact so that new norms reflecting its commitments could take hold. Chaired by an independent doctor, the CIC includes three board members, the CEO, the chief operating officer, the CMO, and five additional medical staff members.

The CIC is responsible for the following:

- Promote awareness and support for the compact;
- Plan and execute strategies for implementation;
- Plan for communication of stories of success and examples for improvement;
- Review progress, at least annually, and report to key stakeholders;
- Review the compact for revisions with stakeholders and forward recommendations to appropriate bodies;

- Develop measures for successful implementation; and
- Provide a process for receiving and responding to issues.

In February 2013, implementation hit a snag when medical staff leadership got cold feet about living the compact. Their reluctance affected the still-fragile relationship with administration. Implementation slowed. Trustee Sherman reflected, "The hardest thing is to true-up words with day-to-day actions. People are fallible; we all do unhelpful things and it will be tough to accept that some decisions are being made in the best interest of the community. Even 'implementation' is being translated by some as 'enforcement,' and there is concern that the agreements would be used as a hammer. Some physicians in the community believe, 'If you win, I lose'; they simply don't believe there can be a win-win."

In late 2013 the CIC created an implementation plan for the coming year. One of the CIC's roles is to be a resource for physicians and others who feel some element of the compact is being violated. Alan Costic, CIC member and board chair, doesn't see this committee as an arbitrator of grievances but as the last-resort option if no other resource can sort through an issue. "My hope is that the CIC spends

---

Exhibit 7.1 Sample Tenet from Each Part of the Salem Hospital Common Ground Compact

Board Contribution
- Oversight to ensure annual goals are set and progress made to better align physician and management behavior with the compact.

Medical Staff Contribution
- Appoint excellent physicians to the Medical Staff and collaborate with the hospital to develop and retain them.

Joint Contribution
- Collaborate to identify and address recognized community needs.

Hospital Contribution
- Provide high-quality facilities and well-trained staff to ensure reliable, high-quality care for our patients.

Source: Salem Hospital. Used with permission.

---

the majority of its time being proactive, not reactive. That is more the role," said Costic. CIC members will have a special responsibility to communicate openly and helpfully with each other. The group can be a model for the cohesiveness they seek to promote via the compact throughout the organization. Costic, summing up progress to date, commented, "In seven years we are miles down the road relative to where we were. Is the rollout fast enough? Not yet. We need to get success stories—of the compact being helpful and relationships getting better—in front of people. My hope is that as problems are brought to us we, the CIC, work well as one."

Each organization's compact reflects its unique challenges or concerns. Likewise, the processes for implementing the compact have great variability. Salem Hospital's implementation committee, which can serve as a sounding board for any party that feels another isn't living by the compact, sends a signal that it takes the compact—and positive relationships between board, administration, and medical staff—seriously.

COMPACT AS KEYSTONE

In 2014, when this book was written, the implementation of Salem Hospital's compact was getting under way. But that effort isn't the only one redefining the organization's culture. Then-CMO Holloway described it this way: "Our compact is the keystone atop an arch. A lot has gone on here besides the compact to build better relationships. Holding the compact up as 'the stone at the top' are both our shared vision and the growing bench strength of our physician leaders."

Considerable change has occurred at Salem Hospital. Today, many physician-run or physician-organized initiatives support collaboration and significant gains in quality and safety. In part, these initiatives also educate physicians about the broader context in which the hospital needs to make decisions so that their ideas and feedback are relevant and, therefore, can be helpful.

The numerous initiatives include the following:

◆ *Revamped peer-review process.* It took three efforts to get it right, but now it is an effective process. In the first redesign each specialty "did its own thing" without staff support, so there was no standard, medical staff–wide approach. A second redesign replaced that structure with smaller, multidisciplinary committees, but they didn't have structure or support; one case could take years to conclude.

In 2010, the most successful redesign resulted in an oversight committee (the multispecialty peer-review committee, or MPRC), a data committee

Salem Clinic:
1999 Compact Retains Relevance for Group Practice Physicians

As Salem Hospital moves forward with compact implementation, it has a resource to help it succeed. The 60-physician Salem Clinic—the largest community-based, independent practice in the city of Salem—has 15 years' experience with explicit, reciprocal expectations to offer as a model. The physicians, who deliver care at Salem Hospital, are well versed in how living by compact commitments can help dispel mistrust and foster cooperation.

The Clinic's Compact Experience: Increasing Trust and Accountability

When Barbara Gunder arrived at Salem Clinic in 1997, the physician–administrator relationship was not what it is today. Back then this relationship could be characterized as distrustful, dysfunctional, and distant. When originally recruited for the position of chief administrator, she wasn't interested in the role if the group was not willing to develop a clear compact and consistently live it. She reports, "A compact is so fundamental to a high-functioning group that, if the doctors weren't willing to seriously consider this work, I would have looked elsewhere to invest my time and energy." Stepping into the chief administrator role, Gunder started to rebuild trust by focusing the doctors on defining the group's mission and values. She believed that once all doctors were behind a clearly stated mission, an explicit compact could heal relationships and strengthen group cohesion because expectations for all parties were defined and measurable. "The onus was on everyone to participate for the good of their colleagues, the partnership, and our community." Within two years she encouraged them to take on compact development.

Fifteen years since it was written, the original compact (reproduced in the appendix) still guides relationships at the clinic. Reviewed yearly with all partners and senior administrators, it continues to be a successful framework for accountability, both among doctors and between doctors and administration. It is referenced during all performance reviews or disciplinary actions and included in conversations with prospective group members and in orientations. The compact reinforces the culture of accountability that has developed under it by drawing like-minded physicians to the clinic.

These annual compact reviews sustain the mutual responsibility needed for such agreements to have real and practical meaning. With healthy levels of trust and communication between doctors and administration, physicians are not hesitant to point to inconsistencies in colleagues' or leadership's behavior. As a complement to the compact, a corporate integrity policy was established that encouraged all physicians to bring concerns to any board member. Sanctioning direct communication with the board members (all of whom are shareholders) gives the physicians a concrete lever for accountability. With regard to administrators' keeping their compact commitments, Gunder has pride in their track record. "All managers hold themselves to the compact as our way of doing business. It provides our ground rules and we stick to them."

Roy Hall, MD, a partner for 41 years, affirms the compact's role in moving beyond distrust. "Our compact allows us to focus on issues that have to be addressed by removing personalities as much as possible. Also it lifts all boats. All physicians know they are held to the same standards." Gunder considers the compact game changing: "It's not just that it set out expectations and communicates that physicians should and can hold me and my team accountable. It positions administration as an ally, removing us-versus-them thinking. Doctors see administration as having their backs." Consequently, it has reset the culture regarding actions that violate agreed-on standards; these are "easy to deal with," in Gunder's words. "What's expected is set out forthrightly, and it's also clear that unhelpful, outside-the-norm behavior will have consequences."

Salem Clinic has made it a priority to preserve an hour of protected time each week for members to interact as one community. Every Monday, the physicians, administrator, and associate administrators gather at noon. Their focus is clinical or financial and ranges from discussions of critical issues to educational updates. Having this scheduled time helps keep all physicians current (eliminating "no one told me that") and allows physicians and administrative staff to hear about trends together. This face time strengthens the group ethos. While larger practices and hospitals confront much more complex challenges around communication and relationship-building, the group size at Salem Clinic makes possible regular meetings with meaningful exchanges.

The Salem Hospital Compact Implementation Committee

Ian Loewen-Thomas, one of the practice's family medicine physicians, participated in developing the clinic's compact. As a proponent of clear expectations, he also chairs Salem Hospital's compact implementation committee (CIC). In this role, he has the opportunity to build bridges between doctors like himself—used to operating with clear expectations and less wary of administration's motives—and those inclined both to hold onto old behaviors and to be highly distrustful of hospital administration. In his words, "The hospital and doctors are all just learning to have a different mind-set."

At this stage, the hospital's CIC is focused primarily on educating physicians and others about how the compact can help smooth out relationships. As Loewen-Thomas puts it, "The Common Ground compact points people to different lenses through which to view situations that are causing tension or misunderstanding. The compact neutralizes knee-jerk reactions that are likely to be unhelpful." He reports that administration is already more aware of the impact of its actions and the critical need for transparency. For their part, physicians are growing more open-minded about needed changes. Given the history that colors current relationships at the hospital, administration has the heavier "burden of proof" in building trust in the compact as a way of life. Loewen-Thomas noted, "Administration will need to be torchbearers. They have to live their responsibilities and model them for other managers. Physicians will be using magnifying glasses to survey administration's actions. Actions consistent with the compact will establish and help deepen trust."

For any organization to succeed, Loewen-Thomas observes, "Success comes down to how well the parts function together. Any toxicity that creeps in downgrades the ability to get important work done." At Salem Clinic, the compact minimizes friction and keeps all parts humming. At the hospital, the clinic doctors are becoming allies and champions for the success of its nascent compact.

that identifies the specific data needs of each component of the peer-review system, and specialty-specific subcommittees. Peer reviews are consistent, fair, and data-driven. Having physicians decide what data to collect increases support for the collection of information. The tenor of the process is that reviews are for improvement, not punishment. The MPRC chair is a 0.6 full-time-equivalent position and is supported by a full-time staff of six. The board is very supportive of the new peer-review system. Jennifer Williams, MD, who chairs the MPRC, calls all the recent changes positive: "The old compact among doctors was contrary to good peer review, but we're changing that. You have to engage the doctors and help them address their own problems."

- *Committee for professionalism, a standing subcommittee of the MPRC.* Begun in 2013, this committee is responsible for establishing and maintaining a professional environment among medical staff.
- *Medical staff engagement committee, formed by neurosurgeon Maurice Collada.* This committee's mandate is to encourage physician engagement with the hospital. Organizing social events is one approach. Another is developing its own physician-satisfaction survey (with input from a local business school professor). This assessment has been used to measure engagement and identify concerns; the committee is moving toward making it a validated instrument that allows for national benchmarking. The medical staff's "five-star recognition program" is another committee initiative. Modeled on the staff reward and acknowledgment program, it recognizes doctors who are role models, demonstrate teamwork, and go above and beyond for patients. To build bridges with administration, this committee joined with CEO Gruber to begin a "Breakfast with the CEO" program, which involves medical staff in twice-monthly discussions over coffee.
- *Quality operations committee (QOC).* This committee began its work in 2012 using physician-led care-improvement projects. With 22 doctors,

administrators, and board members, the committee has responsibility for prioritization oversight of improvement projects. Several doctors, at the suggestion of consultant Jim Reinertsen, MD, visited McLeod Regional Medical Center in South Carolina and brought back this approach to coordinating improvement initiatives. The majority of the QOC are physicians, who now have much greater ownership of the quality agenda.

- *Anesthesiologist-in-Charge (AIC) program, begun in 2009 to bring order to the perioperative area and improve operating room (OR) efficiency.* Working collaboratively with OR nurse management, the AIC functions as a sort of sheriff regarding OR utilization. According to Matthew Boles, MD, interim vice president for surgical services and a contracted anesthesiologist, "This has radically changed the running of the operating room. This is an instance of working together—riding the wave of 'See, we can make things better working together.'" The hospital pays for one anesthesiologist each day to oversee capacity and needs. Having one anesthesiologist managing OR flow using preestablished criteria is a new model for the anesthesiologists and surgeons. A surgical governance group of physicians and administrators established rules for effective use of this shared resource. Cases are classified as A, B, or C, and everyone accepts the process for dealing with infractions (trying to bump a higher-level case with a lower-tier one). Both surgeons and anesthesiologists find the program helpful and wouldn't return to past practices. The AIC program has increased OR capacity by four hours a day.

- *Physician coalition.* This coalition was created by Claire Norton, MD, to increase physician involvement in changes related to documentation, including the hospital's transition to ICD-10 (latest generation of coding). This group of ten—mostly specialists with hospital privileges—meets monthly to provide physician perspectives on information technology, medical records, and coding issues affecting physicians.

- *Trauma Level II designation.* In 2008, after an 18-month process involving stakeholders, Salem Hospital became a Level II trauma center. This time around, the effort (thwarted 8 years earlier; see discussion earlier in this chapter) was a model of engagement. A task force including 20 physicians surfaced concerns and compiled a rich list of questions for the board related to the Level II trauma designation. When the board was ready to go forward with the designation, this time physicians were supportive.

- *Physician Leadership Council (PLC).* The council has 35 members who meet monthly and includes members of the MEC and section chiefs. The group solicits and resolves concerns, ensuring that problems don't disappear into a black hole. The PLC adopted Lean tools and methods, which are spreading throughout the hospital. It also directs the leadership development effort, called the Physician Leadership Institute.

- *Physician Leadership Institute (PLI).* Since 2009, this institute has played a central role in changing the hospital's culture. Under the auspices of the PLI, national healthcare leaders come to Salem to share how and why medicine is transforming. According to Gruber, "The PLI has opened the door to expose more doctors to the changes happening in healthcare. It is the main driver for educating doctors on the realities in the outside world and changes in health-care happening nationally." For many doctors and administrators, the education gained through PLI is the most powerful shaper of behavior and the source of deeper appreciation for why change is needed. According to Jennifer Williams, multidisciplinary peer-review committee chair, "There is growing recognition among some (due to PLI) that professional autonomy is not the same as individual autonomy." Regarding PLI, an independent cardiologist noted, "For me it was precious—really good for learning how to navigate among different interests."

Marty Johnson, intensive care unit director, spoke to the culture-shifting power of PLI:

> Everything had been physician-based, and in the past ten years there has been evolution to be more patient-based. In part we got there through attrition, in part because of an influx of a new breed, and then the PLI has been huge. This program has convinced others of the importance of standardization and doing what's best for patients. It builds on the incredible importance of data to making care better. More doctors understand they can't be passive but need to be agents of change and, in practicing medicine, have to take into account resources. It helps docs think proactively instead of sitting back and not having a voice. Now that about two-thirds have gone through the program, the norm among doctors has shifted.

The power of PLI in changing physicians' mind-set is due in part to insights gained from hearing expert faculty and in part to a required improvement project of the physician's choosing. Participants come to the first weekend with a project in mind and refine the idea so that, by the end of that learning experience, they have defined some piece of improvement work that they will take on.

AN UNFINISHED JOURNEY

Marty Johnson, MD, summarized the gist of the compact as a two-way deal: "A compact can change views to being more cooperative. It states clear responsibilities to others, not just your own constituents. For physicians, this includes the responsibility to practice to standards and to be evaluated. The board has responsibility to listen to physician voices." Yet, as of this writing, some skeptics at Salem Hospital are waiting to see what the next step in compact implementation will bring—if common ground will be a reality and if all parties will act responsibly and respectfully. A realist, CEO Gruber views it this way: "Now it is too early to declare that the impact the compact has had will be sustained. But, I am reasonably optimistic that in five years one could declare the compact and collaboration have worked and produced real results."

Change is the only constant. With healthcare reform, that seems an understatement. While Salem Hospital leadership is focusing on building sustainable relationships with medical staff, even more change is in the air. In November 2013 the hospital announced that it is actively seeking a strategic partner. It's likely that in 2015 the current stand-alone hospital will be part of a larger enterprise, with implications for medical staff that—at the time of this writing—are not clear. And, regardless of the outcome of affiliation talks, succession planning is under way for the CEO position; very likely, a new leader will guide the hospital on the next leg of its journey.

The possibility of a new hospital partner and a new CEO leads some to wonder how the compact will fare in the future. The involvement of board members from the start bodes well for the hospital's continued commitment to the compact. Their view, according to trustee Driggers, is, "We would not hire a CEO who could not support the principles in the compact." This concept is more than sentiment—the compact includes a board commitment on this matter: "The Board commits to selecting a CEO who supports the compact."

In former CMO Holloway's view, "Our trajectory from here might still be something other than a straight line, but there is every reason to be optimistic." The CIC is up and running. Its members are working on a number of items they call "the Silversin list," which identifies steps to embed the compact. That requires the CIC to work with the human resources department to revamp several key processes, including job descriptions, recruitment, and performance reviews. A review of the compact now opens every meeting of the expanded management group of about 120 people, from executives to front-line supervisors.

Salem Hospital has taken many steps to hardwire meaningful cooperation and respect between administration and doctors. As preparation for the future, there is no better strategy.

SUMMING UP

As hospitals gear up to deliver on IHI's Triple Aim (improve patient experiences, improve population health, reduce cost), function as part of an accountable care organization, or pursue any other strategy to respond to the mandate for reform, the need for physician–organization partnership becomes self-evident. At Salem Hospital, medical staff and administrative leadership are working on a relationship deficit to which both contributed over many years. Their experience moving toward common ground holds important lessons for others:

- Even when each side has hardened in its perception of the other, candor, patience, and a willingness to be vulnerable can help create a different future. A well-thought-out compact process provides a structured way to take steps toward mutual respect and cooperation.
- The compact process must be in a context where both shared vision and physician leadership are addressed. Alone, the compact can't produce meaningful results; it has to be buttressed with effective leadership, and all stakeholders need to be on the same page with regard to the organization's future.
- Board involvement can help to constructively move action forward. Trustees can play the role of honest brokers if a relationship is fractured. At Salem Hospital, having the board as one party to the compact helped medical staff feel confident that administration would follow through on its commitments.
- Although trustees should feel urgency for improvement, they cannot sit in judgment of physicians. They need to invest time to understand how policies affect doctors and how doctors perceive executive actions. An "aha . . . *now* I get it" reaction by one trustee to a physician's concern was a pivotal moment at Salem, opening up new possibilities in this organization's compact process—and in its future.

CHAPTER 8

Peninsula Regional Medical Center: New Compact Strengthens Hospital and Medical Staff Alignment

"Let me get this right," I said to Thomas J. Riccio, MD, immediate past medical staff president at Peninsula Regional Medical Center (PRMC). "Right now Maryland caps payments to hospitals—not just per procedure, as it has done for decades, but for total spending—while doctors are paid in the traditional ways? Isn't that crazy-making?"

"Right on both counts," he told me. "That's why the time we invested in creating a compact is so important. There has to be something that gets us over that hump."

THE CONTEXT

Located in Salisbury, Maryland, PRMC is a fairly typical community hospital. And like every other state, Maryland has to get a grip on swelling healthcare costs. But the strategy this state has pursued sets hospitals and physicians at odds with each other through misaligned incentives.

Maryland's Health Services Cost Review Commission (HSCRC) has set the rates for hospital care for all payers since 1977, when the state was granted a waiver exempting it from national Medicare and Medicaid reimbursement principles. Maryland is the only state to authorize a commission to cap prices per procedure. In 2014, the HSCRC introduced the Global Budget Revenue (GBR) model, which sets a cap on the total resources hospitals will receive, essentially controlling the price *and* number of procedures.

Aside from these unusual headwinds to collaboration, PRMC is similar to many community hospitals nationwide. For this reason, the compact construct, which has helped this hospital and medical staff cope with these misaligned financial incentives, may also be very useful to community hospitals facing less convoluted financial circumstances.

Background

The hospital's roots reach back to 1897. The great-great-grandson of the founding physician is today the president of the medical staff and a practicing emergency department physician. The hospital's primary service area has a population of 165,000. With 288 beds, roughly 300 physicians on staff, and 2,000 births a year, PRMC is the most significant hospital on the Delmarva Peninsula, which lies between the Atlantic Ocean and Chesapeake Bay. Salisbury is at the crossroads of north/south- and east/west-cutting highways. With a population of around 30,000, it is the largest city on Maryland's Eastern Shore. In the past, agriculture was the engine of the local economy. Today it's the poultry industry; Perdue, Tyson, and Mountaire all have a presence in the area.

PRMC is a stand-alone, independent hospital. Maryland's GBR agreements for hospital services have prompted institutions such as PRMC—which are not already part of a large system—to form networks to contract with private payers for regional care contracts, to enhance purchasing power, to pool efforts and experience in population health management, and to share resources to develop care pathways.

The hospital will likely become a part of a network; it has been in negotiations with other institutions on Maryland's Western Shore. Its forward-looking plan involves all local physician entities forming a physician–hospital organization, called a "clinically integrated network." Although this work is still in the planning stage, it is already clear to those spearheading the effort that its success will depend on the close collaboration of community physicians, employed physicians, and hospital staff.

The Former, Unspoken Compact

There is nothing out of the ordinary about PRMC's organizational structure, its medical staff structure, or its DNA as a community hospital. Pre-compact, administrators and medical staff had what could be described as a fairly typical relationship, with the usual background tension owing to their different perspectives, cultures, and responsibilities. This gap was widened by an ex-Marine who served as CEO in the mid-1990s. He had an "either you are on my train or we are leaving the station without you" leadership style. He was not a fan of transparency or physician engagement.

By all accounts, his tenure left scars. Almost 20 years later, distrust still seeps into the current CEO–physician relationship in that some physicians are wary of the power the CEO wields; if a decision is not totally transparent to them, they are quick to be suspicious. Some quirks may be unique to PRMC; at ten thousand feet, however, the view of this doctor–administrator relationship resembles that in most hospitals.

The medical staff is a mélange of independent, contracted, and employed doctors. The hospital employed those who sought that arrangement; it did not intentionally build an employed group as competition for community-based doctors. Some specialists are frequently present and intimately tied to the hospital, but primary care doctors have an infrequent presence on the campus because hospitalists provide inpatient care. Until 2012, the prevailing stance of many doctors was that the hospital was their workshop: There they could ply their craft, heal and comfort the sick, and make a living. As long as nurses and operating rooms were at their disposal, how the hospital fared wasn't on their radar screens.

This former, implicit compact can be summed up as follows: Doctors brought their business to the hospital but weren't expected to care very much about its overall performance—in fact, they were often excluded from real influence in strategic decisions. The executive team, along with the board, called the shots but also carried the burden of making everything work out.

MEDICAL STAFF LEADERS PUSH FOR A NEW COMPACT

One aspect of PRMC's compact story is atypical: the physician-led nature of the dialogue and compact development process. The story involves medical staff members who brought the idea inside the institution to move the culture forward. The results achieved, and how the individuals leading the compact effort navigated there, provide lessons many can appreciate and put to use.

The Need for Change Becomes Critical

Tom Riccio, MD, was the indefatigable champion of the compact work at PRMC. A radiologist who oversaw the compact process during his tenure as medical staff president, Riccio claims that timing had a lot to do with the compact's success; others cite his presidency as one of the stars that lined up to create the opportunity for this work to go forward.

As is true for other institutions, no single, cataclysmic event kick-started the process. When trends, issues, and good timing came together to create a felt need to look at alignment issues and a readiness for compact work, Riccio was the right person in the right place. Eric Weaver, MD, who chairs the physician peer-review committee, says of Riccio, "He saw how the local healthcare arena was changing and the big picture, too. He got it before most that going forward, the hospital and doctors can't live apart. We are symbiotic and we need to deal with that reality."

The Peer-Review Problem

The line between insight and action isn't always a straight one. In 2007, one cardiologist on staff ran afoul of Medicare billing, resulting in a fine to the hospital and a Department of Health and Human Services corporate integrity agreement. All PRMC cardiologists subsequently faced new, strict external peer-review requirements. As then–vice president of the medical staff, Riccio led a new committee—the Physician Excellence Committee (PEC)—to create a hospital-wide, multidisciplinary peer-review process. Peer review would be based on fixed criteria and objectively evaluate the quality of care delivered.

This represented significant cultural change that many doctors opposed. The move away from specialty-based peer review was met with the expected pushback: "You can't know enough about my specialty." A strong sense of interdependency among physicians did not yet exist. Physicians didn't feel accountable for colleagues' behavior. For example, while most felt that the cardiologist who had performed unjustified interventions was wrong, they didn't feel responsible; they generally felt the behavior of one rogue doctor had little to do with them. But, living under the corporate integrity agreement brought a lot of physicians up short. In the words of Chief Medical Officer (CMO) C. B. Silvia, "It hurt our pride." Then the PEC began working and attitudes about accountability began to change.

Riccio and others began realizing that business as usual wasn't likely to continue for much longer. The University of Maryland's health system was moving into the Eastern Shore of the peninsula, and MedStar Health, based in the Baltimore–Washington, DC, area, was encroaching on the Western Shore. The Affordable Care Act was the law of the land. Quality and safety would need to be top priorities. Without hospital backing, some specialists could not continue to practice in the community; the hospital's employment of doctors accelerated, causing concern among independent physicians. It was becoming clear that change was both inevitable and unrelenting, and that a lack of synergy between the hospital and medical staff would harm all parties.

The Reimbursement Problem

Maryland's dual system for reimbursing healthcare—global budgets for hospital care, fee-for-service based on negotiated rates for physicians—puts the hospital and its physicians at cross purposes. Moreover, the community has no provision for shared savings. At this time, physician reimbursement in Maryland is beginning to change. Payers are starting to deny physicians' charges for hospital admissions and the hospital's payments—a departure from the past. This is a start toward more closely aligned hospital and doctor reimbursement.

In Maryland, financing for doctors and hospitals may be misalignment writ large, but elsewhere throughout the United States the challenges are similar. (Large, integrated systems that employ physicians and base their compensation on the same measures that drive institutional income—typically, productivity plus quality metrics—may be the exceptions.) When shared savings programs are inadequate or unavailable, it's harder to get the lift of synergy and cooperation. In these cases, it becomes all the more important that medical staff and their hospital share a common vision of the future and a strong sense of purpose. Absent an overarching destination or "north star," each side naturally defaults to maximizing its own interests.

The Time Becomes Ripe

Before he became medical staff president, Riccio heard Jack Silversin describe a compact as a "written, reciprocal deal." However, he couldn't gain enough support from the medical staff leadership to apply the concept to ease difficult situations, such as a controversial effort to replace hospital anesthesia services. He wondered if his group of radiologists could benefit from written mutual expectations, but he chose not to pursue that path. When Riccio became medical staff president, he was encouraged by the successful redesign of the physician peer-review process and felt even more certain that conversation about a new physician–hospital compact could be powerful and the resulting document useful.

In early 2012, Riccio; Janet Pilchard, then-director of physician relations and medical staff services; CMO Silvia; and several other PRMC physicians attended a presentation by Gary Kaplan, MD, the CEO of Virginia Mason Medical Center. When Kaplan showed the compact his organization had developed, Riccio whispered to Pilchard, "This is what I've been talking about." Pilchard then made it her mission, as she says, "To track down Jack Silversin and see if we can get him here."

In short order, the need to do compact work surfaced at a meeting of PRMC's transformation team, headed by Chief Operating Officer (COO) Cindy Lunsford. The focus of this team, of which Riccio and three other physicians were members, had been to develop the capacity for population health management and to create service lines managed by both a physician and an operational leader. The team had been meeting for six months and the service line work was progressing well, until the job description for the service line medical director was distributed. Riccio knew instantly that what the job description asked—empower physician co-leaders for the service lines—was too far outside the prevailing physician culture to work. At the heart of co-managed service lines was a fundamental mind-set change, from doctors as the hospital's customers to doctors as the hospital's partners. He urged the team to not pursue the service line co-management plan any further until groundwork was laid. He proposed that a process to develop a compact could meet several objectives: educate more doctors about market shifts, serve as a call to action, engage in dialogue to build a sense of interdependency, and put some new rules of engagement in writing.

Lunsford recalls her first reaction to the idea of a compact: "Oh, no—that will slow us down. We've been talking for months about co-management." But she, too, could see that asking physicians to take on the kind of leadership needed for service line co-management was a bridge too far. Everyone on that team agreed to take co-management off the front burner, paving the way for a compact process.

GETTING TO A NEW COMPACT

CEO Peggy Naleppa agreed to Riccio's request to share, 50-50, the funding of a compact development. With co-managed service lines on hold, Janet Pilchard contacted Silversin in April 2012. That summer he visited PRMC and interviewed physicians and executives to assess if they had sufficient interest and will to do the work a successful compact process entails.

The Retreat: A Call to Action

The official launch of the effort was a two-day, off-site retreat that September for medical staff and the executive team. Riccio and others reached out to about one hundred core physicians closely tied to the hospital by the nature of their practice. It was work to turn out physicians, but about half of these "active one hundred" participated. For this group, closer alignment and collaboration with the hospital should not have been theoretical; their livelihoods and the hospital's performance are joined at the hip. Yet, at the start, some had little interest in hearing about market changes and the need for closer collaboration with the hospital. What they knew all too well is that being paid less per patient meant having to see more patients. They felt they had little time for much else.

As a result of Riccio and Pilchard's efforts to get the "right people" there, the retreat was extremely successful. Leaders laid out the new healthcare landscape and where PRMC stood. The conversations were not about a new compact but were designed as a call to action. Unless leaders made the case that the medical staff and hospital needed to share a vision of a collaborative working relationship, no compact would make sense.

Airing slights and other sources of mistrust was also part of the weekend. Chief Nursing Officer Mary Beth D'Amico was surprised at how history undermines cooperation. "Stories live longer than I had imagined. It's hard and frustrating that events from before your tenure continue to tinge how people view the hospital and leadership. Some physicians' views about current leaders were shaped by what happened even before *they* joined the medical staff." As she heard and absorbed what doctors were saying about the past and their current views of administration, she wondered, "How will we ever move to neutral?"

The Drafting Committee

At the close of the retreat and again at the following quarterly medical staff meeting, Riccio asked for volunteers to serve on a drafting committee and was impressed with how many stepped up. To ensure that the drafting group would be representative of the broader medical staff, strategically placed phone calls were made to recruit a few doctors who held "traditional views." In all, 17 physicians were joined by 6 executives to draft a compact.

Doctors Only

Riccio suggested that the physicians on the committee meet first without the administrative members so they could talk candidly and think about what they would like from administration in a more collaborative partnership. Ground rules were few: Conversations would be frank, open, and confidential; and referencing deficits in the system—not referencing a particular person—would be the path to resolution of conflicts.

Physician committee members met three times, each time for two and a half to three and a half hours—a significant time commitment, especially at the end of a workday. The meetings were boisterous yet cordial. Some participants had to come to terms with why doctors needed to care about their relationships with administration. "Tell me again how this affects me?" and related questions were hashed out. The group members had an emotional safety net to say anything and to seriously consider what they needed from administration to engage more fully as partners.

Riccio facilitated these meetings; Pilchard helped plan agendas and handled logistics, ensuring that all meetings were well attended. She felt that holding those first doctors-only meetings worked out beautifully. "The key was doctors' being up front. This had to be doctor led, and it was."

The physicians talked about more than physician–administration relationships; they discussed the context for the compact, the changing healthcare environment, and the physicians' role in future clinical integration efforts. One entire meeting was devoted to completing Gosfield and Reinertsen's (2011) *Clinical Integration Self-Assessment Tool v.2.0* so that the physicians understood, in a very concrete way, where PRMC stood.

Doctors can be impatient when processes involve long discussions. At the initial physicians-only compact committee meeting, one physician brought in a draft proposal that included "getting lawyers involved right now since this was about forming a contract with the hospital to form an ACO [accountable care organization]." Given past history with previous administrations, no one blamed him for skipping right to this conclusion. But the group felt that signing onto a fully baked compact would short-circuit much-needed debate. Riccio stated that bringing in lawyers would derail the compact development process, and all other committee members agreed without reservation. This doctor's concern about the compact's being misappropriated to coerce doctors was, according to Riccio, "a good springboard to start a discussion about our mutual purpose and what vision we wanted to create."

During the initial doctors-only meetings, the committee also had to work through the idea that physicians and administration are interdependent. They spent some time formulating the following vision:

> We acknowledge that we are interdependent and we agree to be mutually accountable to each other, the hospital system, and the patient community. We agree to establish a functioning partnership between all members of the medical staff and the hospital to create a sustainable health care system, providing data-driven, affordable, quality care to our patients and our community.

Doctors and Administrators Draft the Compact

After the third doctors-only session, the group was prepared for constructive conversation with executives and, together with them, drafted a compact. In January 2013, Silversin attended one of the two meetings of the full drafting group. CEO Naleppa showed up at all meetings she was asked to attend, even if she had to cancel something else. CNO D'Amico recalls those meetings this way: "The meetings were intense—about the meaning of words. There was a lot of discussion on both sides on the meaning of each word; because we wanted the compact to be clear, we focused on choosing the right words. Parts of some meetings were painful in that we went line by line, word by word until everyone there agreed."

Compact Approval

By the spring of 2013, drafting committee members were discussing the compact outside of their own meetings. Dr. Riccio, at the request of CEO Naleppa, presented an update on their progress to the board of trustees. The first open meeting to share the compact draft with medical staff and get their input was the March 2013 quarterly medical staff meeting attended by Naleppa and other executives.

The follow-up to that meeting was a town hall meeting in May, to which all medical staff were invited; it was promoted as an opportunity for questions and input. Most of the drafting committee members were on hand to explain their work and solicit reactions. They presented the compact as serving four purposes:

1. To set the direction of travel and a destination for the medical staff and the Medical Center to become an integrated health system
2. To create a framework for partnership relations
3. To establish the rules of engagement for relations between the members of the medical staff and the Medical Center, which will facilitate a smoother transition into the world of patient-centered clinical integration
4. To greatly enhance our ability to compete in a data-driven, value-based world, and ensure a place for each of us in the future

The case was made that the changes in healthcare all point in one direction—the need for much tighter coordination of care and collaboration among physicians and all care providers. Exhibit 8.1 illustrates a few tenets from this physician–organization compact. In this formulation, physicians' and the hospital's unique commitments are identified, along with those commitments that apply equally to both. The full version is included in the appendix.

The Medical Executive Committee (MEC) continued to consider the compact and its implications, from the summer of 2012 until its approval by that body in the summer of 2013. The MEC approved a resolution that requires medical staff to sign off on the compact as a condition of reappointment. Eric Weaver, MD, who chairs the PEC and is a member of the MEC, credits the compact with getting medical staff executives to own, in a more profound way, their responsibility for credentialing, medical staff governance, and peer review.

Exhibit 8.1 Sample Tenets from Peninsula Regional Medical Center Compact

Physician Commitments	Mutual Commitments	Hospital Commitments
◆ Understand the new paradigm that we are being measured and evaluated as an integrated healthcare system and not solely as individual practitioners. ◆ Communicate appropriately to colleagues, the healthcare team and the patient. Everyone should know the plan of care.	◆ Support the vision. ◆ Support educational and training programs.	◆ Respect and appreciate physician contributions. ◆ Promote opportunities for physicians to participate in clinical programs.

Source: Peninsula Regional Medical Center. Used with permission.

AN INCREASING SYNCHRONICITY

To underline the purpose and meaning of the compact, the September 2013 quarterly medical staff meeting opened with a YouTube video demonstrating 32 metronomes moving toward synchronization (KickAsshTv 2012). Seeing this phenomenon—independently ticking metronomes begin, in short order, to move as one—drove home the point that much-needed alignment in the organization was possible. At PRMC, clinical integration is defined as "coordination of patient care actions through collaboration to deliver cost-effective patient care." Coordination across a continuum of services requires alignment—which *can* be achieved.

In the summer of 2013, a dozen medical staff members participated in a Transforming Health Care book club. This proved to be an effective way to raise staff members' awareness and knowledge of the issues the institution needed to address. As a result of the discussions, several changes were suggested and then implemented to improve patient care. The focus of the needed changes included revising preadmission testing for procedural outpatients, operating room turnover times, and the admission and discharge process; and expanding evidenced-based pathways across the continuum of care.

Executives and physicians were working in closer collaboration by the second half of 2013. Although all executives use the compact to deal with challenges, the process itself was largely responsible for the shifts in their relationship with medical staff. COO Lunsford commented, "Just having gone through the process, the tone of conversations between administration and physicians is absolutely different. At difficult points we can now negotiate our way through them. It feels so much less adversarial."

New Conversations and Greater Ownership

Evolution in the Medical Staff

Significant is the fact that the doctors took the lead in recalibrating their relationship to the hospital and its challenges. Even if not every physician on staff can cite the compact or even explain what it is, the process changed a core group. Medical staff members, especially those whose livelihoods depend on the hospital, cooperate among themselves more than before; they are stepping up in constructive ways. After the compact process, some made a 180-degree turn; they ask more questions and are less defensive. Hospitalist Chris Snyder, PRMC's chief medical informatics officer and chief quality officer, observes that the more challenging physicians have become allies: "More physicians are becoming the solution rather than presenting problems." He offers examples of physician engagement with improvement work at PRMC that would have been unlikely before the compact process:

- A surgical services operations committee is working on efficient use of the operating room.
- General surgeons are looking at cost per case at the individual surgeon level to find variation and identify standard approaches to minimize variation—with significant buy-in to the project.
- Doctors are volunteering to participate on a discharge operations committee and an admissions operations committee.
- The way physicians and nurses do patient rounds is changing, including more team-oriented rounds with physician-led development of care plans and improved communication with bedside caregivers.
- Providers are engaging in the intake process of patient care plans (providing key information) to help define expected length of stay and working diagnosis.

Physicians are now more engaged in hospital safety. The nurse executive leads a daily safety huddle to review the past 24 hours and what floor staff can anticipate over the next 24. Before, nursing and operational leaders had largely conducted this activity, but now the CMO attends every huddle, and, increasingly, physicians are choosing to participate. PRMC also runs a STAND (situational team analysis debriefing) process whenever there is a near miss or patient harm incident. As soon as possible, the key individuals who were involved meet to review what happened. In the past, the physicians' usual stance was, "Why are you calling a huddle on my patient?" That kind of defensiveness is becoming less common; physicians are more aware of how the whole system, including their behavioral interactions, affects patient care. D'Amico says she recognizes how far they've come when outside doctors express surprise about the STAND process while regular medical staff see it as routine.

The compact conversations have led to several other key evolutions. For one, the medical staff have become less wary of employed physicians. As an example, an employed hospitalist wanted to serve as a medical staff officer. In a departure from the past, the nominating committee put her name forward, reasoning that it was important to recruit officers with talent—and that employment status was no barrier.

Riccio believes the principles in the compact have permeated thinking and language. "Here at PRMC, we now routinely use the words *engagement, empowerment, responsibility, accountability,* and *expectations of performance and behavior.* I hear this language at committee meetings held by the PRMC staff and at the various medical staff meetings and committees. This is our new language, and that's highly significant."

Evolution in the Hospital

The executives I interviewed acknowledge a significant transformation in their approach to working with medical staff. CEO Naleppa makes a point of encouraging her team to use the compact as a moral compass. Lunsford comments:

> We used to feel that we don't want to bother the physicians because of their busy schedules. But that only led to getting too far down a path before checking things out with them. I assumed that they wanted me to do all the background work before reaching out to them. I have learned differently. They are busy and have limited time, and I have learned to set up the conversation differently and more succinctly to involve them in the *decision* phase—not after putting the whole package together.

That mind-set shift matters. Naleppa recalls how master of health administration training programs in the 1980s and 1990s expressly taught aspiring managers to keep physicians at arm's length and to hold information in confidence. The pattern of deciding and then checking it out with stakeholders is not just deeply ingrained, but also reflects the reality that engagement can be messy. To counter that issue, Naleppa is building structures to ensure physician input. As a direct result of the compact, she created a strategy planning advisory committee of ten physicians to weigh in on key decisions.

Eric Weaver, chair of peer review, is a contracted pathologist who provides service to other hospitals in the region. In his perspective, hospitals that don't have a compact *may* talk of transparency, but they (may) involve doctors in strategic planning only because they've been told that they have to. The commitment—on both sides—isn't there for real, ongoing engagement.

Hitting the "Go" Button

To Riccio, the most concrete manifestation of how far the medical staff and hospital have come in two years is the response to reinstituted service line co-management. After having hit the pause button to do the compact work, this work is back on track. Riccio notes:

> The service line change is truly a big deal. It rearranges the traditional departmental structure that physicians are accustomed to. We all see this as a way to get out of silos, strengthen engagement in pathways, and reduce cost. We've had great success with oncology, which has been in place for a year. The medical director position is not honorific in nature—instead, the position is a powerful tool to achieve even greater physician engagement. These individuals will have a contract with performance goals. On so many levels, this is a significant change.

Some service lines have received multiple applications for the medical director position—a good indicator of a different mind-set about accountability and shared responsibility for the hospital's success and the quality of care provided. At PRMC, the unifying concept has recently become, "What's good for the patient?"

More than one person commented that it was good the work was done mostly in 2012. Time and experience have allowed trust to germinate and a different language to take hold. With the launch of Maryland's GBR model, the pressure for change has now been ratcheted up. Meeting challenges wrought by this new payment model without having strengthened the physician–hospital relationship would be more difficult. Mark Edney, chief of surgery, felt that success was in part facilitated by the timing's being right and by judicious use of individuals who had social capital. He commented, "Better to get this hashed out before—*not* in the heat of the moment. It would be a mistake to do this under pressure when it's every person for himself."

ONGOING CHALLENGES

For this community hospital, the physician-led compact work brought a greater sense of "we're in this together." The compact is in its early days, and there have been many perceived violations of it. For the most part, the physicians regularly bring up when administration isn't keeping to its end of the deal.

After the compact was signed, PRMC was hit with a significant budget shortfall and needed to cut $4 million. CEO Naleppa feels that once words are committed to paper, the challenge is in interpretation. "Physicians are quick to point to violations. We all put our own mental models to the words. For budget-reduction meetings, we did brief medical staff officers confidentially—because of privileged information. But to the vast majority of the staff, it looked like the old days of exclusion." She goes on to say, "Without a compact, the world is much more variable. With it, you still need to expect it will be two steps forward and one back. Physicians will have different interpretations and will want to see consistency in administration's behavior." The budget shortfall resulted in some contentious decisions, including closing the Transitional Care Unit. In one meeting a physician vehemently pointed out that, from where he sat, the compact had been violated. A medical staff officer spoke up and said, "You're wrong about that." Crises such as budget reductions can leave scars, but with the compact's having taken root, trust does not go totally off the rails.

At times, the issue isn't interpretation of a phrase in the compact but the fact that physicians weren't included sufficiently early in a decision affecting them. For example, physicians had valuable input to offer about reorganizing spaces on the floors, but their views weren't solicited. When Riccio realized how far along the planning had gotten, he called the executive responsible to the MEC for an explanation. That conversation resulted in the original plan's being scrapped and a new joint physician–administration process going forward.

◆ ◆ ◆

Culture change is a long game. The compact at PRMC has been a much-needed catalyst for doctors and administration to recast their relationship. That the core one hundred doctors now see the hospital's business as their business is a far cry from the recent past. Maryland's GBR initiative is prompting innovation in care delivery. At this writing, a physician–hospital organization is planned. PRMC is pursuing an alliance with similar independent hospitals, with the aim of forming a network. Those structures will only work—that is, deliver on integrated care—if medical staff–hospital relations are constructive. Any suspicion will set back reform.

Surgeon Edney summed up the progress his medical center has made this way: "The instrument of change has been the development of relationships."

After Riccio completed his term as medical staff president, he was invited to sit on the institution's board. Summing up how the compact connects to the challenges he sees looming from his seat at the board table, he comments, "The compact prepares us for this moment."

SUMMING UP

In my interview with CEO Naleppa, she shared her conviction that the explicit compact had become a valuable tool. In reflecting on what I had learned about the process that got them there, I suggested to her that dialogue had helped each party see the other in a more generous light. She agreed. Generosity of spirit would be a significant aid to any institution seeking to succeed as healthcare delivery reforms.

Additional points from this case include the following:

- *Having a physician-led compact process,* from beginning to end, played a key part in the compact's success to date and the greater engagement of physicians. The idea was introduced to the hospital's executive by a medical staff officer. At every point, this physician provided visible leadership, and other physicians also took up the cause. Medical staff met on several occasions prior to sitting down with administration so that they could sort though issues relevant to physicians. Logistical backing was provided by a key supporter in the physician services department, whose assistance was invaluable in getting physicians to attend meetings and keeping the process on track.
- *Self-discovery,* as opposed to being lectured to or handed conclusions, is a powerful way to "raise the heat" for change. The Gosfield and Reinertsen assessment tool the physicians on the compact committee used was more helpful to members' understanding of why change was needed than ten PowerPoint presentations. Doing their own assessment allowed the physicians to draw their own conclusions about what would need to change for their hospital and medical staff for clinical integration to succeed.
- Because of the nature of the compact-development process and the time it requires, *it cannot be done well under duress.* If the heat is high—an organization is in crisis mode—neither physicians nor administrators are likely to focus on the seemingly "soft" issues of trust, relationships, and culture change. Many people I spoke with at PRMC noted that having done the work in 2012–2013 eased the challenges they currently face. The general feeling is that

the core group of physicians is now highly engaged in improvement and that relationships with administration are on the right track. Current anxiety and pressures for change might have hindered an open process if PRMC was just starting compact work today.

◆ One ongoing issue, shared with other organizations with whom we have worked, is *getting the balance right between administration's acting on its commitment to transparency and maintaining confidentiality* during an important decision-making process. During discussions of affiliations or mergers, due diligence is typically carried out in a way that respects the privileged information of all parties. These decisions are the ones likely to have an impact on medical staff.

At PRMC, executives confided in medical staff officers who were not in a position to share the specifics of what they knew with their physician colleagues. While seeming to keep physicians at a distance during affiliation talks might present a stumbling block to compact acceptance by physicians, when medical executive members communicate to their (noncommittee) colleagues that they *are* being kept in the loop—as well as why information must be closely held—they counter doctors' perception that administration isn't serious about transparency. With this communication, and with time and experience, trust in administration should deepen.

CHAPTER 9

A Chief Executive's Personal Application of the Compact Construct

ARTICULATING AND AGREEING TO EXPECTATIONS BUILDS TRUST BETWEEN INDIVIDUALS

My work experience in England dates from 2001, when Jack Silversin and I were asked to provide training and consulting services to the agency created to help modernize that country's National Health Service (NHS). That led to other opportunities to talk about doctor leadership and the compact construct. One individual we met and for whom we subsequently worked is David Flory, CBE, who from 2002 to 2007 was the chief executive of the Strategic Health Authority (SHA) in the North East of England.

At that time, England's Department of Health provided budgets and oversight to NHS organizations through its regional structure of 28 SHAs. Until the Department of Health dismantled the SHAs in March 2013, Flory and subsequent North East SHA leaders used the compact construct to clarify expectations between themselves and NHS organization leaders, which included the executives of primary care organizations, acute care and mental health hospitals, and the ambulance services in this region. Creating reciprocal, clear, and mutually agreed-on expectations between himself and those reporting to him became a hallmark of Flory's leadership style. He credits his use of the compact construct with helping NHS organizations across this region perform better (managing within budget, reducing wait times, improving emergency services), on the whole, than similar organizations in other parts of England for more than five years. (For his services to the Department of Health, Flory was awarded the title Commander of the Most Excellent Order of the British Empire [CBE] in 2009.)

While he was the chief executive of an SHA, Flory operated as the Department of Health in the region; and although the chief executives of the NHS organizations had dotted-line responsibility to him, they also were accountable to their own organizations' boards. Beginning in 2004, the Department of Health created a pathway so that organizations that showed good performance could earn their autonomy and function without any direct reporting line to the Department of Health. In the North East, the majority of these NHS Trusts converted to Foundation Trusts, and the dotted-line authority Flory had had was erased. After that, the relationship between the Foundation Trust chief executive and Flory was defined by influence and mutual dependence—and clear compacts proved valuable.

◆ ◆ ◆

In the spring of 2013, we spoke with Flory in his London office when he was chief executive of the NHS Trust Development Authority, which has responsibility to support all trusts in England to meet criteria for foundation status. He reported that the compacts he created with other leaders in the North East were a significant reason why those organizations were able to achieve results that they and others on the national scene did not think possible. Early in his tenure as chief executive of the North East SHA, he realized that the formal power and role of the SHA would get him only so far in affecting performance across organizations. He understood that the region's NHS organizations were mutually dependent and that the SHA's effectiveness in improving performance across the region depended on cultivating an ethos of collaboration and cooperation—not competition—among the key players.

The potential that clear and reciprocal expectations could have to foster constructive relationships was immediately apparent to Flory when he first heard us speak about our experiences of compact development in US hospitals and medical groups. He says,

> I appreciated how making an explicit deal with another executive could benefit us both. The beauty of a compact between individuals who are mutually dependent to achieve some aim is that it allows for accountability, builds trust, and enhances predictability. Part of the deal I made with the other executives on our patch was that, if you can't deliver on a commitment, I expect you to ring me. Eliminating late-in-the-day surprises engendered trust and cooperation. Developing those bonds of trust is essential because, invariably, things do go wrong. With enough trust, setbacks are seen as that—temporary diversions that can be righted, not proof of insincerity or manipulation.

Asked to specify how a compact between individuals can enhance trust and cooperation, Flory offers, "Trust building comes down to (1) getting clear on the compact between yourself and someone else on whom you are depending for results, (2) doing all you can to deliver on your own promises, and (3) being willing to be challenged if a commitment you made is not being delivered or is perceived by the other individual as falling off the radar."

Flory found that working this way brought out the best in him and the executives he depended on to deliver results. The theme of trust resurfaced many times in our conversation. He said, "You can only be the best you can be if you trust others." He concluded our interview by saying that, in his experience, crafting compacts with others on whom he depended to deliver results "lifted us up."

THE TAKEAWAY

If the timing isn't right to undertake a process to create an explicit physician–organization compact or one between leaders and the organization, you can still form extremely useful compacts between yourself and other individuals.

David Flory's story is that of an executive doing what is within his control: appropriating the concept and applying it to build relationships where such are critical to successful outcomes. When individuals realize they are interdependent for success, a clear statement of commitments—both ways—with accountability builds trust and supports the work that needs to be done.

Part III

MOVING FORWARD:
LESSONS AND GUIDES

Ten Key Lessons from the Cases

All the compact stories in the previous chapters begin with urgency for change or a felt need for a different dynamic between physicians and their organization. Most often, no single incident served as the wake-up call; rather, a constellation of trends, shifts, imperatives—some nuanced, others sharp-edged—fell into alignment to create a *readiness and desire for change* among at least some key players.

That is perhaps the most important lesson of these cases.

Jack Silversin and I have derived several other important lessons from observing, and at times playing an active part in, the processes that these compact participants experienced and managed. Some lessons relate to needed preconditions, some to managing the compact-creating process itself, and others to the outcomes.

1. COMPACTS MUST BE ALIGNED WITH A VISION FOR THE FUTURE

A shared vision is necessary to provide context for the compact. Without agreeing on—and writing down—what you're trying to do *together*, the compact doesn't make sense.

A compact represents agreements, so the obvious question is: agreements around what? Some organizations put time into developing a shared picture of the future as part of the compact process or alongside it. Others craft a compact preamble that lays out the case for clear, reciprocal commitments and use this effectively to set the context for the compact commitments. If the stage is not set by first defining what the doctors and organization are both committed to—or clarifying the shared destination or purpose for making agreements—change is harder to make.

2. THE COMPACT'S POWER TO IMPROVE RELATIONSHIPS LIES IN THE PROCESS TO CREATE IT

Through the process to create a compact, both physicians and administrators look at their own part of the current dynamic and accept new, explicit responsibilities. A common theme among those interviewed is the extent to which relationships in their institution were changed through the dialogue, face-to-face meetings, and sharing of perceptions that are part of compact development. The written agreements are important for hardwiring new behaviors, but without the conversations, the agreements would be powerless to effect change.

These conversations were often very emotional and could be cathartic; people openly expressed loss over what was changing or let go of unhelpful past feelings. Cerebral discussions ("We'll do this if you'll do that") weren't sufficient when old or current feelings were blocking trust and stalling forward movement.

Everyone Must Change

Compact development is an "all change" effort. If approached as "let's get the doctors to change," it will fail. In the stories of successful compact change, administrators also had to look at their own contributions to old, unsuccessful dynamics and be willing to alter their mind-sets and actions.

"Our Compact Is Our Rules of Engagement"

A compact sets out expectations for how people will treat each other to make the organization healthier, to make it capable of change, and to improve patient care. Individuals with successful compact experiences understand from the start that the purpose is to *build a different relationship* and is distinct from the legal imperatives and parameters set forth in traditional contracts and bylaws.

Using a Skilled Facilitator Creates Psychological Safety and Supports Candor

To create psychological safety for all parties, it helps to involve a skilled, neutral facilitator or to engage internal consultants or human resources staff to help set and maintain ground rules for meetings. In some cases venting emotions, particularly frustration and loss, is an important early step in the compact process. If physicians have strong feelings about the loss of their old deal, psychological safety becomes even more important. For participants to be vulnerable enough to share emotions, they need to feel that whatever they say will be respected, not denigrated or used against them. The use of a facilitator creates a protected arena in which such strong feelings can be safely aired.

Building Trust Is Necessary for an Effective Compact and Takes Time

Compact development is one of those activities where "the journey is as important as the destination." The process cannot be rushed. Trust *has* to be built. Time is needed to get genuine buy-in from a critical mass of physicians, administrators, and executives; there are no shortcuts. Every organization featured in this book devoted considerable time to compact development. For most, it took about a year to progress from initial conversations to a finalized document.

During the Process, Ongoing Communication Is a Must

Because developing a compact is likely a months-long process, regular communication about the ultimate goal and the stages of the process is critical. Managers and doctors need information about progress if they are to stay engaged over the long haul. The chief medical officer and CEO can send updates via existing channels, such as newsletters or e-mail. The steering committee might choose to publish print or electronic compact-process updates. If visibility is not maintained, participants may wonder if the initiative fell off leaders' radar screens.

3. LEADERS PLAY CRITICAL ROLES AS SPONSORS AND VISIBLE SUPPORTERS

As the cases in this book illustrate, the compact idea can be introduced by an individual or individuals at any level in the organization. But unless the idea gets the support of executive leadership, it won't have the significance needed to be taken seriously. Senior leaders can't just say that developing a new compact is important; they have to demonstrate through action—showing up at meetings, making resources available to support the process—that they are 100 percent behind the effort.

As part of any compact work, leaders need to be vulnerable to hearing how they are perceived. If they are judgmental toward physicians, cynicism and negativity will erode trust. Again, the two-way nature of the dynamic comes into play; executives and managers have to look at how they knowingly and unknowingly foster physician behaviors that damage relationships, patient care, or the business—and stop enabling such behaviors.

Leaders with a Clear Purpose

In these successful cases, the leaders had a solid understanding of what the compact process was intended to accomplish. They appreciated what a new compact would mean for both physicians and administration. At one institution, leaders took several months to educate themselves first so they could be prepared to lead in new ways.

Engaged Boards

Boards played a key role in some compact journeys. In one hospital, the compact explicitly includes the board and defines its role in improved hospital–physician relationships. As healthcare delivery organizations become more complex through mergers and acquisitions, boards' responsibilities expand. Fiduciary duties, once seen as primarily keeping the organization in the black, now include oversight of quality of care. A key influence on care quality and patient experience—both important to a healthy bottom line—is the quality of the physician–organization relationship. Therefore, every board should embrace oversight of that relationship as a fundamental duty.

Leaders as Active Participants

In these success stories, leaders accepted their primary role in creating a new compact. Although every organization asked our firm for help, our on-site presence varied depending on the ability of internal consultants to do some of the work. In essence, Jack Silversin advised leaders so that *they* could be front and center. This "teaching others to fish" approach meant that leaders felt comfortable enough with this new concept to lead and actively participate throughout the process.

Competent Internal Staff

In the larger organizations presented in the cases, capable in-house staff supported the process. Having some bench strength in the form of physician relations or human resources staff who understood the culture-changing nature of compact work and therefore the need for thoughtful conversation was very helpful. These individuals added value by being credible and able to constructively challenge doctors' thinking. Because multiple meetings spread over perhaps a year are necessary for widespread involvement, understanding, and ownership, it's critical to have staff who can organize logistics, keep the process on track, and give senior leaders honest feedback about the process's timing—and, sometimes, about how inconsistencies in their own behavior are thwarting trust and credibility.

4. BUSINESS-LITERATE PHYSICIANS ARE HELPFUL TO SHARED VISION AND COMPACT WORK

Most of the organizations included in the cases explicitly connected the changed healthcare landscape to the need for deliberate compact work. In making the case for change, they shared market and financial data so that physicians could see what executives see: the challenges on the horizon or at the door. One CEO said, "I'm convinced if the medical staff were looking at the same data that I'm looking at, they would essentially make the same decisions I've had to make."

Expanding doctors' understanding of what's keeping administrators up at night was helpful to the change in some organizations. Some administrators enhanced physicians' understanding by presenting data at a kick-off retreat and at subsequent small-group meetings. One organization not included here ran an early-morning education series for chiefs and managers to give them an in-depth appreciation of the drivers of the institution's economic performance. Salem Hospital makes available annually to medical staff a sophisticated four-part development program that brings in nationally known speakers to share data, trends, and innovations in care delivery.

5. NEGATIVE JUDGMENTS AND STEREOTYPES ARE DEAD ENDS FOR THE PROCESS

One all-too-human tendency creates or exacerbates difficulties in our dealings with others: our inclination to view "them" as the source of whatever's not working, while ignoring our own contributions. Placing responsibility "out there" can derail the relationship building that, at the core, is what the compact is about.

Where the CEO was a physician, there was less "us versus them" in the compact conversations we helped guide. Physicians did, in several examples, have to get beyond distrust of or skepticism about administration. Because it is so essential to a healthy and constructive process, this point is worth underscoring: *Moving beyond negative stereotypes or judgments is necessary for the compact work to have any meaning.* Doing so is not easy. If the dynamic is such that an organization is considering doing compact work, there are likely some critical judgments going both ways. What helps is not casually deciding to trust, but thoughtfully considering how everyone has contributed to the current dynamic or situation. The breakthrough is seeing one's own responsibility and being willing to take the step that upends the current, unhelpful dynamic.

6. PERCEIVED FAIRNESS IN DECISION MAKING IS CRITICAL TO ACCEPTANCE OF RESULTS

In a number of compacts, organizations committed to employing principles of fair process in making decisions that affect medical staff. Everyone wants the playing field to be level—it's a prerequisite for committing to and engaging in any cause. Perhaps because so many physicians feel battered by forces outside their control, interactions that are less than transparent raise their suspicions. Time and again, when physicians co-create a compact, they want the application of fair process to be an organizational responsibility.

The fact that a compact is *reciprocal* bolsters perceptions around fairness. In my observation, this reciprocity greatly helps make an explicit compact attractive to physicians. In contrast to a code of behavior that spells out "thou shalt," a compact balances "gives" with "gets" and reinforces the message that organizations and doctors—in partnership—have responsibilities to each other.

7. A WRITTEN COMPACT FOCUSES AND STABILIZES BEHAVIOR CHANGE, WHICH CHANGES CULTURE

In some parts of Virginia Mason Medical Center, the compact work was referred to as "our cultural revolution." When done well, a clear compact can begin a culture-change process. Writing agreements in behavioral terms, or developing a companion document with examples of behaviors consistent with compact tenets expressed in general terms, gives all parties a clear idea of expectations.

As new behaviors become normative, outliers become obvious. To the extent that the compact represents "the way we do things"—and behavior outside the agreed-on principles triggers consequences (even if just feedback)—the culture shifts. The organizations that created compacts and live by them reported that the culture is different today, especially with regard to physician autonomy. Peninsula Regional Medical Center, which did this work only in the past few years, has experienced a meaningful shift in the degree to which physicians see their own interests and the hospital's as interrelated. For that organization, this shift is already a noticeable and positive change.

At every organization I visited, physician leaders reported that having written commitments to point to in performance-related conversations makes feedback easier to give and more constructive. As one leader said, "Our compact reframes feedback from 'I'm coming down on you for something you did' to 'Let's look at the agreements you committed to.'" The specificity of new expectations supports all parties to engage in different behaviors. The compact isn't a philosophy; if well crafted, it identifies behaviors that are expected—which is how a compact helps shift the culture.

8. A COMPACT ENGAGES PHYSICIANS WHEN IT SPEAKS TO PATIENT CARE

Appealing to physicians' clinical mind-set—putting patients first—was helpful in a couple of compact change efforts. Leaders built the case for a new compact on care, service, and efficiency improvements *for patients*. When leaders talked about the new compact, they emphasized that the reasons for living by it are directly related to improvements in patient care.

9. IMPLEMENTATION HARDWIRES COMMITMENTS INTO POLICY AND PRACTICES

A leader in one organization reported that "the real work begins when the ink on the document dries." Unless organizations make a conscious effort to use the compact and adjust hiring, performance management, and other policies to reinforce it, it will fade into irrelevance. Conscious efforts to implement compact tenets serve as a bridge between "talking about" an explicit deal and the new deal becoming a way of life.

Build New Human Resources Practices

In each case, the organization took steps to integrate its compact into human resources practices. Most organizations used new compacts to recruit and orient managers and physicians or providers. Integrating expectations into performance management and annual reviews further embedded the compact into the organization's fabric—and supported culture change.

Hold Others Accountable

Compact agreements won't have "teeth" if there is no mechanism or tradition of holding the parties to account. For physicians to delegate meaningful authority to their leaders is outside the traditional medical culture. The physician–leader role must include holding others to standards and ensuring quality of care, which is a seismic change both in mind-set and skill level. To foster more effective physician leadership, most organizations discussed in this book invested in selecting and developing leaders willing to accept accountability as part of their role.

Not everyone can adjust to changed expectations. Individuals who choose not to live with the new expectations—after having been given every opportunity to do so—put the compact effort at risk. Leaders who give them a pass are sending the message that "leadership isn't all that serious about new ways of working."

Embed Mechanisms for Reciprocal Accountability

One post-implementation issue that some organizations struggle with is identifying ways to make accountability reciprocal. Important to lasting viability is physicians' sense that they have some mechanism to hold administration to account for its commitments. The general feeling among those I interviewed is that accountability is often asymmetrical: It's relatively easy for the organization to review physician performance and mete out consequences, but the "who" and "how" of holding the organization to account are more ambiguous. At least two organizations systematically ask physicians if they feel the organization is upholding its part of the deal.

One medical group encourages physicians to bring concerns directly to the shareholder board; in one case, the board is a party to compact agreements.

Organizations must find ways to ensure that accountability, like responsibility, flows in both directions. This action helps to reinforce everyone's sense that their compact is fair.

Give Physicians Genuine Authority

When compacts are successful, physicians are active players who have real authority to make decisions and influence their practice environment. They are seen as influential, trusted partners and not rubber-stampers of others' decisions. Their sense of their ability to affect change is what makes physicians constructive partners.

Have the Organization Provide Ongoing Opportunities for Authentic Engagement

Physician engagement has to become a way of life if the benefits of compact work are to be realized. In none of the cases discussed did engagement fade out once the compact was written. If it had, the compact would have become meaningless. Across many organizations, a core tenet of the new compact is the exchange of reduced autonomy for a greater voice in decisions that matter to physicians. A commitment to give physicians greater influence has to be followed up with clear opportunities for authentic engagement, not "Let's give the doctors their say then do what *we* know is best."

10. SUSTAINED OVERSIGHT IS ESSENTIAL TO SUSTAINED RESULTS

After compact implementation, ongoing oversight is essential to the compact's success. The basic model underpinning most quality-improvement work is the plan-do-study-act cycle: Plan a change, implement it, monitor progress, and modify the change as new knowledge about its impact is gathered.

In our model (discussed in Chapter 2), assessment and remediation are the "study" and "act" elements in the cycle. Organizations that successfully did the work years ago ask themselves: Does our compact need to change? Is it still working for us, or have changed circumstances made it important to revisit our vision and original compact?

THE BOTTOM LINE

Among the most critical lessons extracted from these cases is that crafting a new compact shouldn't be done casually or with less than full support of executives. Developing a compact is time-consuming and requires resources to staff and carry out properly. Courage to hold all parties accountable post-development is absolutely essential.

The bad news is that there is no shortcut or work-around to address challenges that stand in the way of care, safety, and value improvement. The good news is that rewriting an outdated compact, in genuine partnership with physicians, offers a sustainable approach to successful organizational change.

CHAPTER 11

Beginning Your Compact Work: A Guide

This chapter builds on the template for compact work described in Chapter 2 and offers a primer for those who want to take the next step and consider or plan a compact process. Whether you are an executive with authority and resources to sponsor the work or a middle manager or physician leader who can generate interest among others, these suggestions and questions can serve to start conversation or as a guide to begin work.

STEP 1: BRING THE IDEA INSIDE AND SHARE IT WITH OTHERS

A compact change process starts by exploring the fit between the current physician–organization compact and the challenges the organization has to address. Questions and considerations include the following:

- What would you say is *your own* unspoken compact with your organization?
- How would you describe the current physician–organization compact? What do physicians expect from the organization? What does the organization expect of physicians?
- What was the compact in this organization ten years ago? What proportion of physicians still expect the old deal but are being asked to engage in changes outside their original understanding of what they signed onto?
- Why does the idea of an explicit compact have appeal for your organization? What do you see and hear (or not see and not hear) in this organization that

makes you think explicit, reciprocal responsibilities for both physicians and the organization would be helpful?

◆ Is the timing right to investigate this idea? Is the need urgent? What other significant changes are around the corner? Given the answers to these questions, is there sufficient bandwidth to take on an effective compact process?

◆ Who else needs to be on board before any compact work could happen? Who's in a position to share that work with those individuals? How can the idea of exploring the current compact and developing an explicit new one be positioned so that these key individuals will be open to learning more about it?

STEP 2: NAME THE PROBLEM(S) A COMPACT MIGHT ADDRESS

If there's sufficient "pull" to go further, you'll want to have a good grip on why you're doing this and the link between challenges you need to address and the current physician–organization compact. At this stage, explore through conversation and succinctly identify the rationale for compact work.

◆ What is the specific reason for developing an explicit physician–organization compact? What challenge does the organization now have that the current compact either contributes to or impedes progress on? How is the current compact related to this problem or challenge?

STEP 3: CONSTITUTE A CORE WORKING GROUP

Logistics for doing the work vary depending on the organization's size and complexity. In smaller organizations, all physicians and managers can meet in one place at the same time. In larger organizations, two distinct groups might have to be organized to carry out the drafting, dialogue, and feedback process.

1. **Core working group:** a group small enough to meet frequently that takes leadership for the compact effort and ideally includes C-suite representation, a human resources executive, and physician leaders. Members of this working group design a process, develop drafts, lead conversations, solicit input, plan for implementation, and modify plans as needed. This group is the sponsor of the compact work.

2. **Ambassadors and supporters:** a larger group, broadly representative of the organization, who spread the word, are champions for the work, and give feedback about the process to the core working group. Some organizations call this the "guiding coalition." Individuals in this group get early exposure to the idea of the compact as well as the rationale for doing this work (the case for change).

Considerations to guide the formation of these two groups include the following:

- Who should be included in the **core working group** that will lead the process?
  - Who needs to participate for the process to have credibility?
  - Which few additional individuals would contribute important views and are independent thinkers, not pushovers?
  - Does the core working group have balance in its representation (e.g., primary care/specialty care, geography, newer organization members/long-termers)?
- Given your organization's size and structure, would a group of **ambassadors or champions** be helpful?
  - Who should be in this group? Consider opinion leaders, those who have helpful expertise, and those likely to obstruct if excluded.
  - If people in your organization don't like the term "ambassador," choose another relevant term (e.g., steering group, guiding coalition, advisory council) that signals to them the group's purpose—that is, its role in supporting or championing the process.

STEP 4: VISUALIZE A DIFFERENT FUTURE

This step has three parts. Begin with assessing whether enough trust exists to have healthy conversation. Then consider if sufficient shared vision is present to fashion a meaningful and useful compact. Last, visualize what a new relationship will require and draft a compact.

Enough Trust to Be Candid

What if lack of trust is a problem that a compact could help solve, yet that issue barricades the way to developing one? It may take a series of facilitated meetings followed by individuals' committing to new behaviors to reset perceptions of trustworthiness.

- Do key players have the capacity for open conversation? Is there sufficient respect and trust among those who need to be involved for conversations to be open and honest? If not, what steps would help all parties resolve old issues?
- If particularly contentious issues need airing, would an outside facilitator be best equipped to design and carry out a process to move toward resolution? Consider using the perceptions activity described in Chapter 12.

Shared Vision

In its most basic form, a written compact puts into words the relationship needed to achieve a shared aim, or vision. It spells out what the parties expect of each other to move toward a state both want to reach. It's not a legal document, but it captures what people of goodwill are committing to so that the relationship between them is conducive to their mutual success. For a compact to have meaning, its promises must not be made in a vacuum but must be connected to a shared future to which there is deep and broad commitment.

- What is the shared vision for the organization? Do executives and managers agree on this? Would most physicians say there is a vision they understand and share and, if so, do they describe the vision in a similar way—or are they working toward some different future vision? Do you know—or is it unclear—how much *any* vision is shared across the organization?
- If a lack of shared vision impedes progress on important initiatives, should time be devoted to a process of creating one? Why or why not?

Draft Compact

Reciprocity of commitments is key. Keep in mind the purpose is not to create a legal document but to define behaviors supportive of a constructive *relationship*. Strive to create a short list of expectations or commitments that captures what the organization needs from each party.

- In drafting a compact, consider imperatives the organization faces today and may need to respond to in the future. What does the organization need from physicians?

- On the other side of the ledger, what benefits do physicians get by being a part of this organization? What will the organization give to support and enable physicians to keep their commitments?

STEP 5: ENGAGE IN DIALOGUE AND COMPACT RATIFICATION

Plan a process that is as inclusive as possible and will be fair and transparent. Especially if this work is meant to mark a new way of relating, the individuals involved should have a positive view of the process—and not believe that their input will disappear into a black hole, with the resulting document bearing little resemblance to the ideas they offered.

Consider the following to help guide this step:

- Given stakeholders' current understanding about the pressures for change, will the process have to include some education about what is changing in the financing and delivery of healthcare? If so, who needs to know what to be an effective participant in conversations about vision and compact? How can they be brought up to speed?
- Toward the goal of including as many physicians and administrative leaders as possible, what logistics make sense? Do meeting opportunities already exist (e.g., departmental) or will special meetings need to be arranged? When? Where? How many? Will participants be paid for attending meetings?
- How many opportunities for input will be offered? Will a second round of comments to a revised draft be sought?
- How will those who are involved be kept abreast of how their input affected the process or was incorporated into the final compact?
- What approval or ratification process is appropriate given your organizational structure and governance? What body or bodies need to approve the final version of the compact?

STEP 6: IMPLEMENT THE COMPACT

Most organizations can take advantage of potent "levers" to ensure their compact becomes and remains a living document. This step usually gets serious attention only after there is a written and agreed-on final compact, but thinking about it as the development phase winds down is important. If there's no capability or will to implement a proposed element in the compact, seriously think about omitting that element. Three levers for implementation are the following:

1. **Outreach, promotion, visibility:** Get the word out and give the compact visibility: Talk about it, write about it in newsletters, and post it in appropriate spaces. Begin medical staff and manager meetings by reviewing the compact. When leaders talk about the compact in formal and informal settings, its relevance is underscored.

2. **Human resources policies and procedures:** Modify human resources policies and practices to reflect the compact. Ensure the modifications apply to executive, managers, and physicians alike.

    ◆ **Policies:** What policies must be changed to reflect the new compact?

    ◆ **Recruitment:** How can the compact be used during recruitment of executive leaders, managers, physicians, and trustees to ensure the best fit of new members with the organization's expectations?

    ◆ **On-boarding:** What opportunities are there during the on-boarding of members to embed the compact? Who are the pivotal influencers on new hires, and how can you be assured the messages they send about expectations are aligned with the compact?

    ◆ **Performance feedback:** Do physicians get regular performance-related feedback? What opportunities exist or can be created to incorporate compact commitments into their performance reviews? For executives, physician leaders, and managers, can the compact expectations be woven into any 360-degree feedback they get on a regular basis? How else can they get feedback as to how well they live compact agreements?

    ◆ **Communication:** What are the most credible and important communication tools that can be used to keep the compact visible? What meetings provide opportunities to bring the compact into conversations?

    ◆ **Training and development:** Given what's outlined in the compact, will different groups (executives, managers, physicians) need new skills? What skills are most needed by whom? Given each group's time constraints and preferred learning methods, what modalities can be used to help individuals develop skills?

    ◆ **Job descriptions:** What amendments need to be made to job descriptions to reflect the new compact?

    ◆ **Acknowledgments and rewards:** Are there currently recognition or award programs into which modeling compact behaviors can be incorporated? Is there any opportunity to tie individual or group bonuses to compact behaviors?

3. **Leaders' actions:** The most potent signal of a different relationship with physicians is the behavior of trustees, executives, and managers. While all parties need to live their agreements, administrative leaders' actions will be under a microscope, and physicians tend to withhold their full support until it is evident that others are taking the compact seriously.

STEP 7: ASSESS AND REMEDIATE

After implementing a compact, keep it vital by monitoring whether it's helping or not. If it's not, determine the reasons and address whatever issues are eroding its usefulness. Some issues to think about as you prepare to assess progress include the following:

- Do senior team members understand how the compact is viewed throughout the organization—which parts of it are working and which are not? If senior leaders are too removed, how can they get an assessment?
- Does the board appreciate that the physician–organization relationship affects care and is within its purview to monitor, along with financial performance, quality, and safety?
- Regardless of how data or comments are collected, do the executive-level leaders have the will to respond to legitimate concerns that are surfaced?

Compact work is best planned and carried out as a group activity, not a solo sport. Here is a final thought as you consider developing a plan or if you have started to put a plan in motion: Create a network for support and sharing ideas. Especially if the idea of administrators' and doctors' getting on the same page is countercultural, those leading the effort should enlist like-minded individuals who understand and support compact work for ongoing support and conversation. Leaders may face challenges from those who think, "Let's not rock this boat." The best life jacket you can pack is colleagues who are up to the adventure and willing and able to be mutually supportive in both smooth and choppy seas.

CHAPTER 12

Questions from the Field:
Jack Silversin Responds

No one has had more experience than Jack Silversin in advising healthcare organizations on how to most constructively use a physician–organization compact as a tool to build physician engagement in organizational challenges and to help change cultures. In response to frequently asked questions, he shares his observations and insights from more than 30 years of doing this work.

Question: *I'm the chief of an internal medicine department, not the CEO. What should I do if I think our unspoken compact keeps us stuck?*

This is the most common concern I hear after making presentations about the compact. A leader—physician or administrative—in the middle of the organization sees the need but on his or her own doesn't have the authority or status to do anything about a new compact, while top leaders' own actions contribute to an unhealthy dynamic with physicians. Your challenges are sharing the idea in a way that allows senior leadership to see the situation as you do and presenting it as objectively as possible. Success calls on practicing the art of managing upward. Even if, in your view, leaders' attitudes or behaviors are part of the problem, you'll need to put any judgment aside. Your communication won't be effective if others get the sense they're being criticized or indicted.

First, whom do you need to influence and what's important to them that the current compact thwarts? The compact idea has to be shared in terms that senior leaders not only relate to but also view as important to their work or goals.

Second, in sharing the information, keep in mind that someone other than you may be the best messenger. Think about who is in the best position—is credible to and has respect of those you seek to influence—to talk about the compact. Put aside your ego and be strategic. In my experience, executives who are not physicians are more receptive to an idea such as this when it's presented by someone who's not only trusted but is also a member of the same "tribe."

If, for whatever reason, timing isn't right or top leaders either can't hear the message or won't agree to sponsor the work, you still have a few options:

- One, share the idea with colleagues—physician and administrative—to broaden their understanding of how chipping away at the old compact with requests for change amounts to loss in physicians' eyes. That insight alone can be very useful to those who sponsor change, expect physicians to be excited and get on board, and then are frustrated when engagement is less than needed. If they understood that some changes are adaptive, they might approach the change project differently. When the change involves physicians and is adaptive in nature, their having a voice and an active hand in crafting the solution are key.
- Two, develop a department- or program-specific compact. While it won't be as helpful as an organization-wide new deal, it can help the physicians and your administrative colleagues work together to make faster progress on changes that are called for. A compact might be a practical way to get everyone on the same page and lay the foundation for greater two-way accountability—you and other leaders to department members, and them to you. Your department's progress might draw the attention of other leaders and stimulate conversation across the organization regarding how a broader new compact can help accelerate the institution's work.
- Last, there is always the option to do as chief executive David Flory has done (see Chapter 9) and clarify mutual expectations whenever you are working collaboratively with colleagues. Ensure you share the same end point or aim, then spell out what you will be accountable to each other for as the work progresses.

Question: We don't trust them and they don't trust us—how do we start?

I see this all the time—if there were a good working relationship, it's highly unlikely either party would be looking to develop a different compact. The organizations I work with typically are experiencing some challenge and have the courage to ask for help. Lacking trust, it's unlikely either party will be up for any open and truthful conversation. I spoke in the Netherlands where a chief executive commented that he personally would find such open conversation with physicians too threatening. Clearly, he had anxiety about the possibility. But I wondered how it could be less threatening to him and the organization to avoid reality and allow negative emotions to fester.

The only thing worse than hidden agendas and overt sabotage is when a group of people agree just to get along. Doing so allows them to nod in agreement to a condition or behavior they know they won't abide by once the conversation ends and they walk out of the room. That further undermines trust. When lack of trust presents a barrier to real engagement and candid conversation, I deal with it first.

One approach I frequently use asks both sides, or groups, to come together for half a day to share perceptions and unpack contributors to the current dynamic. This perceptions activity begins by dividing participants into their natural grouping (i.e., physicians or executives), during which time they answer three questions within their group and then share answers in a large-group discussion:

1. How do we see ourselves in this relationship (our contributions, strengths, and shortcomings)?
2. How do we see you (contributions, strengths, shortcomings)?
3. How do we think you see us?

After hearing what one group has to say about the other, each asks questions to better understand how their behavior accounts for others' perceptions. Because it touches on identity and negative perceptions, the activity needs to be carefully structured and skillfully facilitated. Setting and enforcing clear ground rules creates enough safety for people to first write their responses and then candidly discuss what they wrote. The activity helps clear the air of old baggage and perceived slights so that, at the conclusion of the activity, any commitments made are more likely to be kept.

The main takeaway from the activity is for each side to understand and own their responsibility for the unhelpful perceptions others formed of them. Then, appreciating that behavior and actions are messages that others interpret, accurately or not, each party identifies a few behaviors they will consistently follow to change old stories and negative perceptions.

Whether it's this facilitated and structured discussion or a series of meetings to air differences and move forward, this is tricky work and has to be expertly conducted. If we could just wave a wand and dispense with unhelpful attitudes of others, life would be so much easier. But, like a truth-and-reconciliation process, giving each group the opportunity to hear why others hold the perceptions they do—what they have done or currently do that leads others to see them as they do—is part of the healing process. Through this activity, I've seen real transformations in how people view each other. When we understand the reasons an individual or group took some particular action, our perception of them expands. If people can hear how they're seen, accept their own responsibility for what currently is, and commit to doing things differently, even unhealthy relationships can get on a better footing. The prognosis for moving on is correlated with each group's knowing and acknowledging, at least to themselves, that their own success depends on their taking actions that build trust. People discover the power to be successful is in owning what they do that undermines the relationship. A friend once put it this way, "You can get to be right or you can have the relationship!" And that's as true in business affairs as in personal life.

Question: We're a large organization with employed doctors, community doctors, and contracted doctors. Can a compact work for us?

I'm frequently asked whether employed doctors and voluntary medical staff should be held to the same compact. In my view the answer, for the most part, is yes. One common set of expectations across subgroups of medical staff is helpful—it reduces complexity and speaks to a level playing field. You don't want to set up a situation where different doctors are held to different standards of behavior. In reality, a community hospital, for example, is a resource for the benefit of the whole locale, and every doctor—regardless of his or her affiliation with it—is responsible for behaving in ways that ensure high-quality, safe care and the hospital's long-term viability.

That said, I have worked with organizations in which it was important to include a couple of compact tenets applicable only to employed doctors. Being an employee may bring unique or additional responsibilities—for example, having an annual performance review. When that's the case, the rationale for different or extra compact expectations has to be explicit, make sense, and not be perceived as conferring advantage or creating an unfair situation relative to others (e.g., access to patients, opportunities to serve on the board or committees).

Question: This system has multiple hospitals and several clinics, and its service area is extensive. Should we still try to create and live under one compact?

Compact development is easier and more straightforward in smaller organizations or ones with few sites, but I've helped with the compact process in very large, multi-site organizations and it can work in those, too. A single compact makes sense if, across the system, there is a shared identity and common vision as one entity with multiple sites, versus strong local institutions stitched together to create a system in name only. Having a single set of expectations for administrators and physicians, regardless of where they practice, works to deepen their identity as a system.

There are three important issues to consider when working across sites:

1. *Representation:* Forming an ambassador group or guiding coalition in addition to the core working group will be necessary. Both groups should reflect the diversity of the whole organization. That is important for three reasons:
   - Participation in compact dialogues will be greater if a few people from each local site are active proponents who encourage others to get involved. Familiar faces have more credibility than those from a central office or distant site.
   - If both groups are broadly representative of sites that have their own local color—issues, challenges, cultures—the final document is likely to reflect as many parts of the organization as possible and therefore will resonate with those across the different sites.
   - Communication from the center to the parts will be facilitated if there are representatives from each location to spread the word, provide updates, and keep the flow of information back to the center open.

2. *Communication:* Ensure that a mechanism is in place to keep everyone informed throughout the process, which may take many months, especially in a complex, geographically spread organization. Those who assemble and give feedback early in the process may assume the whole compact initiative is over and their feedback made no difference if they don't get regular updates on how the work is going.

3. *Standardization:* Consistency of message across sites is critical. Meetings should be organized along similar lines and, as much as possible, be run in the same way. I encourage the use of a standard agenda; standard presentation, if one is part of an introductory meeting; and standard format and meeting length. Depending on how different or unique local sites are—an extended-care facility is unlike a primary care clinic—there may be opportunities to customize some messages, but the key "what we're doing and why" should be consistent. Sticking to the script as much as possible ensures the core message is delivered to all stakeholders in the same way. It reduces variability across sites that could lead to misinterpretations and confusion. I also recommend standard communication—in message and format—when it comes to explaining the final compact and why some suggestions are incorporated and others are not.

Question: Is the compact only for doctors or also for our physician assistants (PAs) and nurse practitioners (NPs)? They practice alongside us, so shouldn't they be included?

For me, it all goes back to the early step, "identify the problem you are trying to solve." Is the underlying issue that physicians aren't aligning with the organization's change agenda? Is it more broadly that providers are not as willing to give time to process improvement as other staff members? What is the reason for doing compact work in the first place? That's the first consideration.

For all the reasons this book has explored, the physicians' compact/psychological contract is most resistant to change, and physicians are central to the organization's ability to meet quality, safety, and efficiency goals. Providers who are not physicians are growing in stature and importance to care delivery, so this is not to diminish their professional status; but I don't think that they are as deeply imbued as physicians are during their training with the message that they have an inherent right to certain entitlements and can expect to be their own bosses. I have been challenged by those who are upset about singling out doctors for compact work. When they ask, "Are doctors really different?" my answer is, "Yes . . . *different*, not *better*."

The inclusion of advanced-practice clinicians such as NPs or PAs or even optometrists depends on how they are used and perceived in your organization. Where physicians view them as colleagues and the culture values egalitarianism, excluding them could be destructive to the culture that already exists. In some organizations, NPs and PAs share all responsibilities with physicians with the exception of taking call. I recommend including other providers when there's good reason to and when excluding them would rupture relationships that are currently functional and collegial. The TCP-ThedaCare compact is an example of one inclusive of all providers.

Question: You talk a lot about fair process. How is that connected to the compact?

Fair process is a way of making decisions that my clients find helps to address a perceived loss—namely, influence over issues of importance to physicians. Not that long ago, doctors exercised significant influence in the organizations in which they practiced. Administration and the board viewed them as primary customers and saw meeting doctors' needs as a key part of their job. You can find senior members of hospital medical staff who talk about those times as the golden age.

Today, patients and their families are hospitals' primary customers. Given the pressure and urgency for improvement, management can no longer cater to the individual needs of doctors and, for their part, doctors haven't been willing, or able, to agree with each other when asked for input. Managers avoid physician involvement, which means decisions don't take advantage of physicians' expertise and perspective. This situation alienates physicians and reduces their willingness to collaborate on important issues.

From surgeons booking operating room time to children kicking a soccer ball, we are all wired to want and expect fair play. A significant literature exists around the concept of procedural justice. It points to the reality that we will accept a decision, even one we disagree with, *if* we think the process that led to the decision wasn't political or corrupt but was based on merit or credible data and was transparent—that is, fair. So applying principles of fair process helps doctors re-engage. And acceptance of the decisions is greater when physicians and others view the process leading to them as transparent and objective.

A process for soliciting input into a decision can be both efficient and fair if these steps are followed:

- Clarify the criteria that will be applied to making a decision.
- Invite input in the context of the criteria.
- Decide.
- Provide an explanation for the decision that includes how doctors' input shaped the final decision.

Question: How do compacts affect how doctors collaborate with and treat each other?

Some compact elements may apply to individuals' actions (e.g., treat everyone with respect), while others are achieved only through physicians' working collectively in new ways (e.g., coordinate and integrate care). I have often commented that the changes needed for physicians to work differently with colleagues, decide on best practices, and give feedback to and hear feedback from each other are huge. Physicians on one "side" of a compact aren't monolithic. They represent a wide diversity of views, needs, and generations. Some may have very different economic interests than others. These factors tend to make collaboration among doctors every bit as challenging as building a cooperative partnership with management.

Question: So, if this is about a relationship between physicians and an organization, who is the "organization"?

The leaders are the proxy for the "organization" in compacts that name it and physicians—or providers—as the parties. But each organization should decide who *exactly* is covered by that term—who is accountable to the physicians or providers to live up to that side of the compact. Executives and middle managers? Does it include branch, site, or departmental leaders? This decision needs to be made and communicated so there's no ambiguity about it—for the sake of accountability and the compact's usefulness.

Whenever physicians accept a formal leadership role and are paid for their administrative time to achieve agreed-on goals, they are part of management/administration. That means it's incumbent on physicians in these roles to live by the organization's commitments as well as the physicians', a reality that is easily overlooked or can be uncomfortable for physician leaders. They might feel caught between furthering the organization's agenda and being ostracized by colleagues. Physician leaders who attempt to promote change are too often labeled as having gone to the dark side, which speaks volumes about the legacy compact ("our leaders are supposed to protect us") and the extent to which it operates.

It should be clear by now that a compact triggers many changes and, to succeed, it can't exist in isolation but must be supported by additional development opportunities or initiatives. When any compact states "physicians delegate authority to leaders" or has language to that effect, I recommend that those empowered leaders—if they don't already know how—learn to use colleagues' input in decision making. We have to move away from management's opinion that if "you talk to one doctor . . . you've talked to one doctor." When a physician leader commits to an administrative colleague that the department will do X, his or her word needs to be good—the agreement can't be hollow; it can't mean "I'll do my best." And that's only possible if the department has truly authorized its leader to act on its behalf—and getting members' input prior to committing to administration is key to physician leaders' success.

Question: *Someone I know said her organization wrote a compact and it's made no difference at all. Does it fail as often as it works?*

A compact isn't for everyone—it's a transformational change. Some organizations have a history of implementing the "change du jour" and will reach for any new management fad that seems promising without doing the real work of recalibrating this all-important physician–organization relationship. I'd say that most often, a new compact makes no difference when the people bringing it into the organization treat it as a technical change when it is adaptive. After writing all the nice-sounding words, senior leaders and managers continue with business as usual and don't reflect compact commitments in their day-to-day behavior or way of thinking. Also, physicians don't stretch and adopt new behaviors, and aren't held accountable for not even trying.

There are plenty of reasons that, once developed, the compact doesn't provide benefits—but a major one is failing to see how deep and fundamental the changes really are, for everyone. The simplicity of the compact idea is both an asset and a liability in that it seduces leaders into thinking "here's a remedy." But what many don't understand is how profound the changes embedded in the compact really are.

Question: The compact makes so much sense, but are there situations for which you don't recommend it?

A new compact is not a panacea, and in certain circumstances I'd emphasize that it's not the right thing to do. Here are a few.

First, if big change is in the air and it's not likely the present organization will be in a position to keep promises, then don't start this work. If you're on the cusp of a major transition—merger, acquisition, executive shake-up—that will change priorities or result in a reorganization, put off this work. Likewise, crises related to financial loss tend to wreak havoc emotionally and cause distraction. If significant losses are about to be reported or a turnaround firm is at the door, anxiety will be running high, so don't embark under those conditions. When there are just too many pressing priorities that demand leaders' time, a compact is unlikely to get the attention it needs.

If there is no structure, mechanism, or intention to hold physicians accountable, it would be pointless to engage people in developing a compact. A compact doesn't have to be deferred until physician leaders have completed training that provides needed skill and insight; it's not uncommon for physician leadership development to go hand-in-hand with compact development. But the *will* to hold everyone—including physicians—to account for living by compact agreements has to be present.

Question: This work sounds so serious—do you recall any lighthearted moments during the compact development process?

Oh, certainly. I feel tremendous joy in seeing things work out, in helping people mend fences and move forward together. On a light note, the word "compact" clearly has a few meanings—and both cynics and supporters have made fun of all of them over the years.

In one organization the people I worked with habitually referred to our activity as "compacting." So there were compacting meetings and compacting documents. During this assignment all I could envision was the mechanical process of crushing and squeezing that an industrial or kitchen compactor does—not a very helpful image. But for whatever reason the term worked for that client, and as far as I know, no one there rejected the idea—or the relationship building it fostered—because of it.

At one organization undertaking compact work, a physician leader always joked that a meeting with me was time to pull out his makeup kit and powder his nose—the word brought to mind his mother's old-fashioned makeup compact. Despite the ribbing he gave me, he got the point of the work and changed along the way. Near the end of our compact work, he and I had a meeting with the chiefs reporting to him and he handed each a simple compact case that opened up to reveal two mirrors. He did it as a joke, but the meeting turned to the metaphor of the two mirrors and how important it is for leaders to see not only themselves clearly but also how they interact with others—to observe their own actions or attitudes that contribute to all the dynamics around them.

VIRGINIA MASON MEDICAL CENTER PHYSICIAN COMPACT

Organization's Responsibilities

Foster Excellence
- Recruit and retain superior physicians and staff
- Support career development and professional satisfaction
- Acknowledge contributions to patient care and the organization
- Create opportunities to participate in or support research

Listen and Communicate
- Share information regarding strategic intent, organizational priorities and business decisions
- Offer opportunities for constructive dialogue
- Provide regular, written evaluation and feedback

Educate
- Support and facilitate teaching, GME and CME
- Provide information and tools necessary to improve practice

Reward
- Provide clear compensation with internal and market consistency, aligned with organizational goals
- Create an environment that supports teams and individuals

Lead
- Manage and lead organization with integrity and accountability

Physician's Responsibilities

Focus on Patients
- Practice state of the art, quality medicine
- Encourage patient involvement in care and treatment decisions
- Achieve and maintain optimal patient access
- Insist on seamless service

Collaborate on Care Delivery
- Include staff, physicians, and management on team
- Treat all members with respect
- Demonstrate the highest levels of ethical and professional conduct
- Behave in a manner consistent with group goals
- Participate in or support teaching

Listen and Communicate
- Communicate clinical information in clear, timely manner
- Request information, resources needed to provide care consistent with VM goals
- Provide and accept feedback

Take Ownership
- Implement VM-accepted clinical standards of care
- Participate in and support group decisions
- Focus on the economic aspects of our practice

Change
- Embrace innovation and continuous improvement
- Participate in necessary organizational change

VIRGINIA MASON MEDICAL CENTER LEADERSHIP COMPACT

Organization's Responsibilities

Foster Excellence

- Recruit and retain the best people
- Acknowledge and reward contributions to patient care and the organization
- Provide opportunities for growth of leaders
- Continuously strive to be the quality leader in health care
- Create an environment of innovation and learning

Lead and Align

- Create alignment with clear and focused goals and strategies
- Continuously measure and improve our patient care, service and efficiency
- Manage and lead organization with integrity and accountability
- Resolve conflict with openness and empathy
- Ensure safe and healthy environment and systems for patients and staff

Listen and Communicate

- Share information regarding strategic intent, organizational priorities, business decisions and business outcomes
- Clarify expectations to each individual
- Offer opportunities for constructive open dialogue
- Ensure regular feedback and written evaluations are provided
- Encourage balance between work life and life outside of work

Leader's Responsibilities

Focus on Patients

- Promote a culture where the patient comes first in everything we do
- Continuously improve quality, safety and compliance

Promote Team Medicine

- Develop exceptional working-together relationships that achieve results
- Demonstrate the highest levels of ethical and professional conduct
- Promote trust and accountability within the team

Listen and Communicate

- Communicate VM values
- Courageously give and receive feedback
- Actively request information and resources to support strategic intent, organizational priorities, business decisions and business outcomes

Take Ownership

- Implement and monitor VM approved standard work
- Foster understanding of individual/team impact on VM economics
- Continuously develop one's ability to lead and implement the VM Production System
- Participate in and actively support organization/group decisions
- Maintain an organizational perspective when making decisions
- Continually develop oneself as a VM leader

(continued)

Educate

- Support and facilitate leadership training
- Provide information and tools necessary to improve individual and staff performance

Recognize and Reward

- Provide clear and equitable compensation aligned with organizational goals and performance
- Create an environment that recognizes teams and individuals

Foster Change and Develop Others

- Promote innovation and continuous improvement
- Coach individuals and teams to effectively manage transitions
- Demonstrate flexibility in accepting assignments and opportunities
- Evaluate, develop and reward performance daily
- Accept mistakes as part of learning
- Be enthusiastic and energize others

VIRGINIA MASON MEDICAL CENTER BOARD COMPACT

Organization's Responsibilities

Foster Excellence

- Facilitate the recruitment and retention of superior board members
- Provide a process for regular, written evaluations and feedback through annual board self-evaluation
- Support governance excellence with adequate board resources

Listen and Communicate

- Share information regarding strategic intent, organizational priorities and business decisions
- Offer opportunities for constructive open dialogue
- Report regularly on implementation of strategic plan and achievement of specific board objectives
- Disclose to and inform board on risks and opportunities facing the organization
- Provide materials to members necessary for informed decision making sufficiently in advance of board meetings

Educate

- Provide information and tools necessary to keep members informed and educated on local and national health care issues
- Provide educational and training opportunities to maintain a high level of board member effectiveness and knowledge

Lead

- Manage and lead organization with integrity and accountability
- Create clear goals and strategies
- Continuously measure and improve patient care, service and efficiency
- Resolve conflict with openness and empathy
- Ensure safe and healthy environment and systems for patients and staff

Board Member's Responsibilities

Know the Organization

- Know the organization's mission, purpose, goals, policies, programs, services, strengths, needs
- Keep informed on developments in the Health System's areas of expertise and on health care policy and future trends and best governance practices

Focus on the Future

- Spend three-fourths of every meeting focused on the future
- Consistently maintain a current and vital strategic plan

Listen and Communicate

- Actively participate in board discussions
- Participate in educational opportunities and request information and resources needed to provide responsible oversight
- Provide and accept feedback
- Represent the board to the organization and be an advocate for the organization in the community

Take Ownership

- Attend meetings
- Ask timely and substantive questions at board and committee meetings consistent with your conscience and convictions
- Prepare for, participate in, and support group decisions
- Understand and participate in approving annual and longer range financial plans and Quality and Safety oversight
- Make an annual, personal financial contribution to the organization according to personal means
- Serve on board committees or task forces

Promote Effective Change

- Foster innovation and continuous improvement
- Pursue necessary organizational change

THEDACARE PHYSICIANS—THEDACARE COMPACT

Preamble

Our vision is to be the most sought-after health care partner creating measurable, world-class quality outcomes at the lowest cost. Achieving this vision depends on trusting, collaborative partnerships.

The foundation of this partnership is a set of clearly defined expectations that are mutually beneficial. ThedaCare and ThedaCare Providers are each responsible to hold themselves and each other accountable to the expectations in this compact. This document serves as a framework of needed behaviors and is intended to be adaptable and to evolve over time. Our dedication to continued dialogue is key to making this compact a valuable and useful set of agreements that support our ability to achieve our vision.

Compact

Provider Gives

Patient-centered, customer-focused care

I will provide exceptional service for our patients by anticipating and exceeding their unique needs, especially in an evolving competitive market.

World class quality

I will provide measurable, world class clinical and service quality (≥95th percentile performance) that is visible to patients, employers and our communities.

Collaboration and communication

I will work toward a common vision by collaborating and communicating effectively with patients, team members, specialists, and all parts of our system.

Leadership

I will demonstrate leadership through active involvement at the site, call group, and organizational level.

The Organization Gives

Commitment to primary care and collaborative specialty relationships

While valuing all members of the group, we will build ThedaCare's differential value on the primary care provider–patient relationship model.

World class resources

We will invest in the resources and skills necessary to enable providers to have satisfying careers and achieve our vision.

Collaboration and communication

We will actively involve our providers in shaping strategic, clinical and operational decisions.

Leadership

We will demonstrate leadership by setting a vision that reflects our commitment to lead the market through excellence and innovation.

(continued)

Create a positive work environment

I will model and create a work environment that is open, trusting, respectful and fulfilling.

Flexibility

I will seek new solutions and adopt new practices in order to improve my performance.

Recognition and reward

I will recognize and celebrate the accomplishments of the organization and my team members.

Fiscally responsible

I will manage resources that ensure the best value for my patients and for the organization and its customers.

Create a positive work environment

We will model and create a work environment that is open, trusting, respectful and fulfilling.

Flexibility

We will continuously seek ways to improve how we lead and manage our organization.

Recognition and reward

We will provide compensation and benefits that reflect the group's accomplishments and enable us to attract and retain the best providers. We will demonstrate appreciation and celebrate provider and team contributions.

Fiscally responsible

We will deliver the best value—exceptional quality at the lowest cost for our consumers while exceeding financial targets.

"THE DECLARATION OF INTERDEPENDENCE": STILLWATER MEDICAL GROUP PROVIDER COMPACT

Provider Gives:

Provide patient-centered care and service

Be flexible, willing to change and open to innovation

Be on the team, not above or outside

Stay informed and actively involved

Recognize and support organizational leadership

Be accountable for personal and group results

Be a good steward of organizational and healthcare resources

Stillwater Medical Group Gives:

Provider-directed group practice

Engagement in decision making and fair process

Organizational support and resources to practice best medicine

Fair compensation based on market and group performance

Excellent communication

A COMPACT BETWEEN MEMORIAL HERMANN PHYSICIAN NETWORK AND ITS PHYSICIAN MEMBERS

Preamble

With Clinical Integration, MHMD has introduced a new model of providing care to the Greater Houston community—an interdependent network of physicians that collaborate with each other and the Memorial Hermann Healthcare System to provide better quality, highly efficient, more cost-effective care. The Clinical Integration model demands physician accountability, technology infrastructure, and substantial investments of time and resources by both MHMD and its physicians. Clinical Integration thus enables the delivery of better care by its physicians, leading to collective negotiating with health plans for contracts that return enhanced value to MHMD physicians. The compact that follows identifies a reciprocal set of commitments and accountabilities between MHMD's elected leaders and the physician members. It is designed to support the organization and its members to achieve the MHMD strategic vision and build capacity to respond effectively to future challenges and opportunities.

Compact Attributes

1. Provide Evidence-Based Clinical Care/Governance

Physicians: provide evidence-based clinical care
- Practice according to current evidence and best practices
- Participate in robust clinical educational programs and peer review
- Achieve and maintain competency and board certification
- Meet mutually agreed upon regulatory, quality, recredentialing and safety goals

MHMD: provide excellent governance
- Abide by all tenets of Physician's Commitment in this Compact
- Maintain primary loyalty to the member physicians, nurture their success, and act consistently in their best interests including in their relationships with the hospital system
- Apply current knowledge and relevant best practices to guide contract negotiations and bonus compensation models in a way that is both equitable and that aligns economic incentives to improve care
- Support physicians to become knowledgeable about the issues and trends that will affect our success
- Ensure that effective mechanisms are in place to foster physician involvement in the organization's work and in decisions that affect them and MHMD's success

2. Be Transparent

Physicians: be transparent
- Share with MHMD quality data from my practice on a timely basis
- Disclose interests in entities or activities potentially detrimental to the Mission, Vision, and/or Goals of MHMD

(continued)

MHMD: be transparent

- Use a transparent, criteria-based, fair-process approach for making decisions likely to have significant impact on physician practice and MHMD's success as a physician organization
- Provide timely and clear information regarding all MHMD membership criteria
- Provide timely and clear information regarding all quality performance measures
- Provide timely and clear information regarding all agreed upon benchmarks and scoring criteria
- Provide timely and clear information regarding remediation requirements and procedures
- Provide timely and clear information regarding the status of contract negotiations with health plans, and all resulting contract terms, conditions, requirements, fee schedules, and pay for performance distribution methodology
- Provide timely and clear information regarding MHMD's budget and financial performance

3. Collaborate

Physicians: collaborate

- With physician colleagues and other caregivers to enhance the value of our care
- With MHMD elected leaders by seeking communication, engaging in decisions, and aligning behavior with commitments made by MHMD on their behalf
- With our hospitals to improve the safety and efficiency of patient care
- With health plans to improve care and align economic incentives
- With patients and our community to improve health

MHMD: collaborate

- With physicians to provide up-to-date clinical information, education and decision support that will facilitate the implementation of evidence-based medicine in their practices
- With physicians by providing timely reports regarding their performance on agreed upon quality and efficiency programs
- With physicians to help them achieve quality and efficiency goals
- With physicians by providing services that ease the administrative burden of practice and address their practice needs
- With physicians by providing education and support to help them meet regulatory, quality and safety requirements

4. Demonstrate Compassion and Respect

Physicians: demonstrate compassion and respect

- To better understand experience and perspectives of patients, other physicians and healthcare professionals and MHMD
- To resolve any conflict that may arise in a collegial, effective manner
- To follow the MHMD professional code of conduct in all relationships with physicians, nurses, personnel and patients

(continued)

MHMD: demonstrate compassion and respect
- Create clinical programs that support physicians in all practice settings
- Seek to understand and consider how the organization's decisions will impact on the practice and professional satisfaction of our physician members
- Advocate consistently for physicians in ways that advance the needs and enhance the success of all parties

5. Be Accountable

Physicians: be accountable
- To integrate feedback to improve performance
- To achieve agreed upon quality and efficiency standards, thus promoting the health of the entire Houston community
- To assist colleagues to improve clinical performance

MHMD: be accountable
- Seek feedback from physicians regarding how well the board is meeting its obligations as outlined in this compact
- Provide effective practice management tools to ease the administrative burden of both clinical practice and MHMD's quality performance measures
- Maintain the confidentiality and security of the quality improvement data obtained from physician practices
- Maintain the confidentiality and security of fee information and billing data obtained from physicians' practices
- Provide timely and accurate performance feedback

6. Maintain Professionalism

Physicians: function as a member of the MHMD team
- Participate in clinical committees and leadership development
- Attend and participate in appropriate meetings
- Accept that nonparticipation in these meetings means forfeiture of direct influence on decisions and acceptance of those decisions made by MHMD physician peers

MHMD: foster a team spirit
- Implement approaches to communication likely to engage individual and small groups of doctors, including enabling meeting attendance by electronic means
- Ensure that physician meetings are well planned and worthwhile expenditures of physician time
- Ensure that new members of MHMD receive a robust orientation program regarding our mission, vision, goals and compact
- Create leadership training programs for physicians desiring professional growth to enhance the MHMD vision

(continued)

Physicians: support innovation

- Evaluate and implement evidence-based emerging technology including "cyber connectivity"
- Adapt to more effective ways of practicing medicine
- Exhibit creativity in seeking innovative solutions and new opportunities
- Share best practices with the organization
- Maintain openness and adaptability to change
- Participate in new studies and protocols

MHMD: support innovation

- Set an "innovation agenda" to seek, import and foster the adoption of relevant best practice innovations from within and outside our organization
- Nurture our relationship with The University of Texas Health Science Center at Houston (UTHealth) Medical School to help physicians stay current with leading practice and technology and to enable MHMD physicians to participate in clinical trials led by UTHealth
- Encourage and support MHMD physicians in the evaluation and implementation of evidence-based emerging technology including "cyber connectivity"
- Encourage and support MHMD physicians in adapting to more effective ways of practicing medicine
- Develop and promote educational programs to help physicians maintain best practices
- Encourage MHMD physicians to create and share new ways of working when a significant gap exists between current and desired performance

SALEM HOSPITAL COMMON GROUND COMPACT

BOARD CONTRIBUTION

◆ Oversight to ensure annual goals are set and progress made to better align physician and management behavior with the compact.

◆ Prior to making significant decisions, provide opportunities for Medical Staff physician leaders and Administration to be engaged and have perspectives understood and considered.

◆ The Board commits to selecting a CEO who supports the compact.

JOINT CONTRIBUTION

◆ Collaborate to identify and address recognized community needs.

◆ When competing, demonstrate we are committed to a respectful relationship with your competitors.

◆ Jointly make investments in electronic health records that will facilitate achieving an integrated record that supports sharing information across physicians and settings.

◆ Establish the Compact Implementation Committee with the responsibility of working with physicians, administrators

HOSPITAL CONTRIBUTION

◆ Provide high-quality facilities and well-trained staff to ensure reliable, high-quality care for our patients.

◆ Promote and support the services of credentialed Medical Staff who provide services in the Hospital and whose actions are consistent with the Compact.

◆ Provide the Medical Staff timely, relevant information and engage in meaningful, two-way communication using systems developed by the Medical Staff.

◆ Demonstrate respect and appreciation for Medical Staff contributions. Model

(continued)

MEDICAL STAFF CONTRIBUTION

◆ Appoint excellent physicians to the Medical Staff and collaborate with the Hospital to develop and retain them.

◆ Support the ongoing existence and viability of Salem Hospital.

◆ Develop and use recognized systems of communication to stay informed. Take responsibility for staying informed.

◆ Be respectful and collaborative team members.

- and trustees to achieve the Shared Vision and Compact, balancing what is best for the individual with what is best for our community of professionals and our Hospital.

- Work with the Hospital Administration to develop and maintain modern data systems for the management of our patients.

- Choose leaders who demonstrate ongoing development of technical, interpersonal and leadership competencies necessary to be successful in leadership positions.

- Work with leaders to create a shared structure for effective physician involvement in decisions that impact clinical care and/or are likely to generate strong emotions:
  - Act consistent with decisions made by Medical Staff leaders and Administration and support them, even when it was not the one you preferred.

- Actively engage in quality and resource management to decrease variation from best-known practice:
  - Create physician-led, patient-centered, data-driven standards for quality, service and efficiency.

- Collaborate with the Hospital on assessing and managing financial risk in a changing world.

- respectful behavior, be available to listen and be collaborative team-members.

- Work with the Medical Staff to develop and maintain modern data systems for management of our patients.

- Collaborate with Medical Staff leaders within the shared structure to set and achieve standards for high quality and efficiency.

- Support the Medical Staff leadership in implementing physician-led, patient-centered, data-driven standards and improvements;
  - Support with data systems and reports;
  - Support with staff trained in data analysis and process improvement; and
  - Maintain a process for tracking progress.

- Assist Medical Staff in complying with regulatory requirements.

- Collaborate with the Medical Staff on assessing and managing financial risk in a changing world.

SALEM CLINIC PHYSICIAN COMPACT

MISSION STATEMENT: It is our mission to improve the health of those we serve in a spirit of compassion and respect. To that end, we make the following commitment:

GROUP MEMBER RESPONSIBILITIES

With Regard To Patient Care
- Provide timely feedback to patients.
- Promote physician-to-physician communication where care indicates.
- A priority of every provider will be to see his/her own patients when they need to be seen.
- Provide adequate and timely documentation.
- Work with patients to make them active participants in their health care and to support them to take responsibility for appropriate, cost-effective care.
- Improve quality and reduce cost by decreasing variation through practicing evidence-based medicine.

With Regard To Group Citizenship
- All physicians will exhibit pride in the work environment and demonstrate a positive collegial attitude, which, in turn, will promote respect and partnership among physician staff, support staff and management. All physicians will provide direct and constructive feedback to other physicians and address and resolve conflicts, which may arise.
- Attend and participate in department and group meetings.
- Physicians, support staff and management will respect and follow organizational guidelines and participate in the development and achievement of goals.
- Comply with Corporate Integrity Policy.
- Be flexible for the good of the group.
- Demonstrate courtesy, respect, integrity, and honesty toward colleagues, staff and all of our physicians.
- Accept organizational decisions that are based on our commitment to put the patient first.

With Regard To The Use Of Financial And Other Resources
- Provide adequate and timely submission of charge slips.
- Demonstrate interest in understanding the cost of the care you provide.

WHAT GROUP MEMBERS GET
- Opportunities to contribute to the direction and improvement of our physician-led group through participatory governance (empowerment—a voice in running the organization).
- A fiscally responsible organization.
- Fair market compensation based on work effort and patient satisfaction.
- Accountability from Administration.
- Timely and accurate information that enables physicians to take responsibility for their performance.
- A fair and consistent application of all contracts, policies, compensation, and this compact to all physicians.
- Opportunity for strengths of individuals to be combined with strengths of group membership.
- Opportunity to improve physician education and skills.
- Practice in a group setting that promotes physician wellness.

PENINSULA REGIONAL MEDICAL CENTER PHYSICIAN COMPACT

Vision Statement

We acknowledge that we are interdependent and we agree to be mutually accountable to each other, the hospital system, and the patient community.

We agree to establish a functioning partnership between all members of the medical staff and the hospital to create a sustainable healthcare system, providing data-driven, affordable, quality care to our patients and our community.

Physician Commitments

- Understand the new paradigm that we are being measured and evaluated as an integrated healthcare system and not solely as individual practitioners.
- Communicate appropriately to colleagues, the healthcare team and the patient. Everyone should know the plan of care.
- Adhere to guidelines, standardized protocols, and best clinical practices.
- Maximally utilize IT technology in the management of patients.
- Participate in data-driven quality and utilization management programs.
- All members of the medical staff shall be held accountable for achieving acceptable data-driven results.
- Support and participate in medical center programs and service lines.

Mutual Commitments

- Support the vision.
- Support educational and training programs.
- Support clinical research.
- Respect the authority of our physician and administrative leaders.
- Show physician colleagues, administration, board members, and hospital personnel respect.
- Work together in partnerships to understand and meet patient needs.
- Strive to understand each point of view and proceed with integrity and transparency.
- Hold each other accountable.
- Create and participate in the design and implementation of best clinical practices.
- Should opportunities for physician/hospital business partnerships arise, transparent consultation and mutual considerations shall be pursued.

Hospital Commitments

- Respect and appreciate physician contributions.
- Promote opportunities for physicians to participate in clinical programs.
- Integrate physicians into leadership and management of hospital operations.
- Include physician leaders in strategic planning.
- Support physician clinical decision making and provide timely ancillary services and results.
- Collect, process and distribute outcome data and cost data in an appropriate manner to achieve best clinical practice and patient management.
- Support marketing programs.

References

Argyris, C. 1977. "Double Loop Learning in Organizations." *Harvard Business Review* 55 (5): 115–25.

———. 1960. *Understanding Organizational Behavior.* Homewood, IL: Dorsey Press.

Chassin, M. 2013. "Improving the Quality of Care: What's Taking So Long?" *Health Affairs* 32 (10): 1761–65.

Collins, J. 2001. *Good to Great: Why Some Companies Make the Leap . . . and Others Don't.* New York: HarperCollins.

Consumer Reports. 2013. "How Does Your Doctor Compare?" *Consumer Reports Health: Special Report for Wisconsin Residents.* Special insert (February).

Cutler, D. M., and F. S. Morton. 2013. "Hospitals, Market Share, and Consolidation." *Journal of the American Medical Association* 310 (18): 1964–70.

Davies, H. T. O., and S. Harrison. 2003. "Trends in Doctor–Manager Relationships." *British Medical Journal* 326 (7390): 646–49.

Degeling, P., S. Maxwell, J. Kennedy, and B. Coyle. 2003. "Medicine, Management, and Modernisation: A Danse Macabre." *British Medical Journal* 326 (7390): 649–752.

Edwards, N., M. J. Kornacki, and J. Silversin. 2002. "Unhappy Doctors: What Are the Causes and What Can Be Done?" *British Medical Journal* 324 (7341): 835–38.

Edwards, N., M. Marshall, A. McLellan, and K. Abbasi. 2003. "Doctors and Managers: A Problem Without a Solution?" *British Medical Journal* 326 (7390): 609–10.

Federal Trade Commission. 2014. *Analysis of Agreement Containing Consent Order to Aid Public Comment.* Accessed December 5. www.ftc.gov/sites /default/files/documents/cases/2002/05/pisdanalysis.pdf.

Fisher, R., and S. Brown. 1988. *Getting Together: Building a Relationship That Gets to Yes.* Boston: Houghton Mifflin.

Frey, B. S., and M. Osterloh. 2012. "Stop Tying Pay to Performance: The Evidence Is Overwhelming—It Doesn't Work." *Harvard Business Review* 90 (1–2): 51–52.

Garelick, A., and L. Fagin. 2005. "The Doctor–Manager Relationship." *Advances in Psychiatric Treatment* 11 (4): 241–52.

Goman, C. K. 1997. *"This Isn't the Company I Joined": Seven Steps to Energizing a Restructured Work Force.* New York: Van Nostrand Reinhold.

Gosfield, A. G., and J. L. Reinertsen. 2011. *Clinical Integration Self-Assessment Tool v.2.0.* Published May. www.uft-a.com/CISAT.pdf.

Greenleaf, R. K. 1998. *The Power of Servant Leadership.* Oakland, CA: Berrett-Koehler Publishers.

———. 1977. *Servant Leadership: A Journey into the Nature of Legitimate Power and Greatness.* Mahwah, NJ: Paulist Press.

Heifetz, R. A. 1998. *Leadership on the Line.* Cambridge, MA: Harvard University Press.

Heifetz, R. A., and D. L. Laurie. 1997. "The Work of Leadership." *Harvard Business Review* 75 (1): 124–34.

Heifetz, R. A., and M. Linsky. 2002a. *Leadership on the Line: Staying Alive Through the Dangers of Leading.* Boston: Harvard Business School Press.

———. 2002b. "A Survival Guide for Leaders." *Harvard Business Review* 80 (6): 65–74, 152.

Heifetz, R. A., M. Linsky, and A. Grashow. 2009. *The Practice of Adaptive Leadership: Tools and Tactics for Changing Your Organization and the World.* Cambridge, MA: Harvard University Press.

Hoffman, R., B. Casnocha, and C. Yeh. 2013. "Tours of Duty: The New Employer–Employee Compact." *Harvard Business Review* 91 (6): 48–58.

Institute of Medicine. 2000. *To Err Is Human: Building a Safer Health System.* Report, edited by L. T. Kohn, J. T. Corrigan, and M. S. Donaldson for the Committee on Quality of Health Care in America. Washington, DC: National Academies Press.

Jost, T. S. 2014. "Implementing Health Reform: Four Years Later." *Health Affairs* 33 (1): 7–10.

Kaissi, A. A. 2005. "Manager–Physician Relationships: An Organizational Theory Perspective." *The Health Care Manager* 24 (2): 165–76.

Kane, C. K., and D. W. Emmons. 2013. "New Data on Physician Practice Arrangements: Private Practice Remains Strong Despite Shifts Toward

Hospital Employment." American Medical Association. Published September 17. www.ama-assn.org/ama/pub/news/news/2013/2013-09-17-new-study-physician-practice-arrangements.page.

Kavilanz, P. 2013. "Doctors Bail Out on Their Practices." CNN Money. Published July 16. http://money.cnn.com/2013/07/16/smallbusiness/doctors-selling-practices/.

Kenney, C. 2011. *Transforming Health Care: Virginia Mason Medical Center's Pursuit of the Perfect Patient Experience.* New York: CRC Press.

KickAsshTv. 2012. "32 Out of Sync Metronomes End Up Synchronizing." YouTube video. Posted September 26. www.youtube.com/watch?v=kqFc4wriBvE.

Kim, W. C., and R. Mauborgne. 1997. "Fair Process: Managing in the Knowledge Economy." *Harvard Business Review* 75 (4): 65–76.

Kohn, A. 1993. *Punished by Rewards: The Trouble with Gold Stars, Incentive Plans, A's, Praise, and Other Bribes.* New York: Houghton Mifflin.

Kornacki, M. J., and J. Silversin. 2012. *Leading Physicians Through Change: How to Achieve and Sustain Results,* second edition. Tampa, FL: American College of Physician Executives.

Kotter, J., and D. Cohen. 2002. *The Heart of Change.* Boston: Harvard Business School Press.

Lewis, C. S. 1944. "The Inner Ring." Memorial lecture at King's College, University of London. www.lewissociety.org/innerring.php.

Moses, H., D. H. Mateson, E. R. Dorsey, B. P. George, D. Sadoff, and C. Yoshimura. 2013. "The Anatomy of Health Care in the United States." *Journal of the American Medical Association* 310 (18): 1947–63.

Pink, D. H. 2009. *Drive: The Surprising Truth About What Motivates Us.* New York: Riverside Books.

Plsek, P. E. 2013. *Accelerating Health Care Transformation with Lean and Innovation: The Virginia Mason Experience.* Boca Raton, FL: CRC Press.

Rich, N. 2014. "The New Origin of the Species." *New York Times* Sunday magazine (March 2): MM24.

Rosenberg, T. 2011. *Join the Club: How Peer Pressure Can Change the World.* New York: W. W. Norton.

Rousseau, D. M., and M. Greller. 1994. "Human Resources Practices: Administration Contract Makers." *Human Resources Management* 33: 385–401.

Schein, E. H. 1980. *Organizational Psychology*, third edition. Englewood Cliffs, NJ: Prentice-Hall.

Senge, P. 1990. *The Fifth Discipline: The Art and Practice of the Learning Organization.* New York: Doubleday/Currency.

Simon, D. W., H. H. Brooks, and C. E. Rossman. 2009. "Clinical Integration: A Guide to Working with the Federal Trade Commission to Enhance Care Through Pro-Patient, Pro-Innovation, Pro-Efficiency Provider Networks." Foley and Lardner LLP. Published January 21. www.foley.com/intelligence /detail.aspx?int=9217.

Tichy, N., and R. Charan. 1989. "Speed, Simplicity, Self-Confidence: An Interview with Jack Welch." *Harvard Business Review* 67 (5): 112–20.

Toussaint, J., and R. Gerard. 2010. *On the Mend: Revolutionizing Healthcare to Save Lives and Transform the Industry.* Cambridge, MA: Lean Enterprise Institute.

US Department of Justice and Federal Trade Commission. 1996. *Statements of Antitrust Enforcement Policy in Health Care.* Published August. www.justice .gov/atr/public/guidelines/0000.htm.

Whyte, W. H., Jr. 2002. *The Organization Man,* revised edition. Philadelphia, PA: University of Pennsylvania Press.

Wisconsin Collaborative for Healthcare Quality. 2014. "WCHQ Measures Summary Report." Accessed November 3. www.wchq.org/reporting/wchq _measures_summary.php?provider_id=31.

Suggested Readings

Our application of a compact between doctors and their organizations draws from ideas of social psychologists and change-management theorists. This suggested-readings list points you toward original source material or adjunct material that we found useful in explaining the concept or helping organizations design constructive compact development processes.

BACKGROUND ON THE PSYCHOLOGICAL CONTRACT

Early research into the construct of a psychological contract between employees and employers was done by academics with an interest in industrial and organizational psychology. Three books by investigators of the construct are:

Argyris, C. 1960. *Understanding Organizational Behavior.* Homewood, IL: Dorsey Press.

Levinson, H., C. Price, K. Munden, H. Mandl, and C. Solley. 1962. *Men, Management, and Mental Health.* Cambridge, MA: Harvard University Press.

Schein, E. H. 1980. *Organizational Psychology,* third edition. Englewood Cliffs, NJ: Prentice-Hall.

Change-leadership thought leader John Kotter wrote his Massachusetts Institute of Technology master's thesis on the psychological contract. It was published as an article:

Kotter, J. 1973. "The Psychological Contract: Managing the Joining-Up Process." *California Management Review* 15 (3): 91–99.

A more recent review of research into the psychological contract in work settings is:

Conway, N., and R. B. Briner. 2005. *Understanding Psychological Contracts at Work.* Oxford, United Kingdom: Oxford University Press.

Other authors have written about practical applications of the psychological contract in organizations:

Goman, C. K. 1997. *"This Isn't the Company I Joined": Seven Steps to Energizing a Restructured Work Force.* New York: Van Nostrand Reinhold.

Strebel, P. 1999. *The Change Pact: Building Commitment to Ongoing Change.* New York: Financial Times/Prentice-Hall.

Wellin, M. 2007. *Managing the Psychological Contract: Using the Personal Deal to Increase Performance.* Burlington, VT: Ashgate Publishing Company.

The contemporary authority on the power of unspoken expectations in organizational life is Carnegie Mellon University professor Denise Rousseau. Her extensive writings include both books and articles, such as the following:

Rousseau, D. M. 2004. "Psychological Contracts in the Workplace: Understanding the Ties That Motivate." *Academy of Management Executive* 18 (1): 120–27.

———. 2001. "Schema, Promise and Mutuality: The Building Blocks of the Psychological Contract." *Journal of Occupational and Organizational Psychology* 74 (4): 511–41.

———. 1996. "Changing the Deal While Keeping the People." *Academy of Management Executive* 10 (1): 50–61.

———. 1995. *Psychological Contracts in Organizations: Understanding Written and Unwritten Agreements.* Thousand Oaks, CA: Sage.

Rousseau, D. M., and M. Greller. 1994. "Human Resources Practices: Administrative Contract Makers." *Human Resources Management* 33 (3): 385–401.

ADAPTIVE CHANGE

In working with healthcare organizations, the idea that has the most impact when joined with the psychological contract is that of adaptive change. According to Ronald Heifetz, changes that challenge deeply held assumptions or expectations are "adaptive" and deserve special consideration and approaches:

Heifetz, R. A. 1998. *Leadership Without Easy Answers.* Cambridge, MA: Harvard University Press.

The following book was written as a guide for those responsible for implementing adaptive change:

Heifetz, R. A., M. Linsky, and A. Grashow. 2009. *The Practice of Adaptive Leadership: Tools and Tactics for Changing Your Organization and the World*. Cambridge, MA: Harvard University Press.

The following book sheds light on the risks to those leading adaptive changes and how to successfully negotiate those risks:

Heifetz, R. A., and M. Linsky. 2002. *Leadership on the Line: Staying Alive Through the Dangers of Leading*. Boston: Harvard Business School Press.

Articles in *Harvard Business Review* on adaptive and technical change include:

Heifetz, R. A., and D. L. Laurie. 1997. "The Work of Leadership." *Harvard Business Review* 75 (1): 124–34.

Heifetz, R. A., and M. Linsky. 2002. "A Survival Guide for Leaders." *Harvard Business Review* 80 (6): 65–74, 152.

CORPORATE CULTURE

Edgar Schein has been closely associated with the first use of the term "corporate culture." His insight on behavior inside of organizations remains unmatched in clarity and practicality. The book that directly follows is Schein's classic look at culture inside organizations; the second one is a practical handbook for culture change.

Schein, E. H. 2010. *Organizational Culture and Leadership*, fourth edition. San Francisco: Jossey-Bass.

———. 2009. *The Corporate Culture Survival Guide*, new and revised edition. San Francisco: Jossey-Bass.

More recently, Schein authored two books focused on skills of great value to leaders:

Schein, E. H. 2013. *Humble Inquiry: The Gentle Art of Asking Instead of Telling*. San Francisco: Berrett-Koehler.

———. 2011. *Helping: How to Offer, Give, and Receive Help*. San Francisco: Berrett-Koehler.

FAIR PROCESS

While moving ahead without physician input seems efficient, the fallout can derail any change, including compact implementation. We urge clients to read a classic *Harvard Business Review* article for insight into how an involvement process can be timely, inclusive, and fair:

> Kim, W. C., and R. Mauborgne. 1997. "Fair Process: Managing in the Knowledge Economy." *Harvard Business Review* 75 (4): 65–76.

Kim and Mauborgne's work draws on earlier research and writing in a field first named "procedural justice" by social psychologist John Thibaut and legal scholar Laurens Walker, who concluded that people will accept an outcome that is not in their own best interest as long as they perceive that an impartial and transparent process led to that decision:

> Thibaut, J., and L. Walker. 1975. *Procedural Justice: A Psychological Analysis.* Hillsdale, NJ: Lawrence Erlbaum.

Research findings in this field are reported in:

> Lind, E. A., and T. R. Tyler. 1988. *The Social Psychology of Procedural Justice.* New York: Plenum.

For a summary of the legal and organizational applications of procedural justice, I recommend an excellent review of Lind and Tyler's book:

> Vidmar, N. 1991. "The Origins and Consequences of Procedural Fairness." *Law and Social Inquiry* 15 (4): 877–92.

GUIDE TO CHANGE IN HEALTHCARE ORGANIZATIONS

Last, our previously published book takes a comprehensive view of how to successfully implement change in healthcare organizations affecting physicians:

> Kornacki, M. J., and J. Silversin. 2012. *Leading Physicians Through Change: How to Achieve and Sustain Results,* second edition. Tampa, FL: American College of Physician Executives.

Our website is www.consultamicus.com.

Index

Driggers, Bonnie, 113, 122
Due diligence, 140

Edney, Mark, 137, 139
Edwards, Nigel, 4
Electronic medical records, 70; ThedaCare system for, 50–51
Employed doctors: Silversin on compact tenets and, 168
Employee-generated standards of behavior: at Stillwater Medical Group, 79–80, *81*
Employees: psychological contracts and, xix
Employers: psychological contracts and, xix
EMRs. *See* Electronic medical records
Entitlement, xviii, 22; newer generation of physicians and, xxi; physicians' tacit expectations of, 6, *7*; Salem Hospital physicians and, 108
Epic (electronic medical record software), 50
Ernst and Young, 86
Every-man-for-himself compact: shortcomings of, xx
Executive leadership: sponsorship and support of, 149–51
Explicit compacts: need for, xx

Facilitated adaptation, xxi
Facilitators: skilled, psychological safety and, 148–49
Fagerlund, Shelly, 27
Failure of compact: Silversin on, 172–73
Fairness in decision making: compact acceptance and, 152
Fair process: inclusive, ThedaCare compact and, 55, 64; Silversin on compacts and, 170–71; at Stillwater Medical Group, 77
Federal Trade Commission, 84, 85
Fenn, Scott, 86, 90
Fernandez, Keith, 86, 87, 92, 93, 96, 100
Fiduciary duties: engaged boards and, 150
Fifth Discipline, The (Senge), xxii
Fisher, Roger, 110
Flory, David, 166; personal application of compact construct, 141–43
Foundation Trusts (England), 142
Franklin, Kathy, 52, 54, 55, 62
FTC. *See* Federal Trade Commission
Furman, Cathie, 41

Garrison, Cort, 104
General Electric: compact change and transformation of, xx
Gerard, Roger, 52
Getting Together (Fisher and Brown), 110
Glenn, Michael, 35, 36
Global Budget Revenue (GBR) model (Maryland), 125, 126, 137, 138
Gogola, Jon, 93, 97
Good to Great (Collins), 73
Gosfield, A. G., 132, 139
Greenleaf, Robert, 60
Greller, Martin, 4
Griffin, Shawn, 92, 96
Gruber, Norm, 105, 106, 107, 108, 111, 114, 119, 121, 122
Gruner, Dean, 54, 60, 67
Guiding coalitions: definition of, 159; multisite organizations and, 169
Gunder, Barbara, 117, 118

Hall, Roy, 118
Hallett, Mark, 63, 64
Hanson, Dan, 27
Harvard Business Review, xx, 55
Healthcare Effectiveness Data and Information Set, 50
Healthcare industry: seismic shifts in, xvii
Healthcare reform: physician employment and, 47–48; physicians as linchpins of, xvii
HealthPartners (Minneapolis), 69, 75, 80; Lakeview Health System's merger with, 77, 82
Health Security Act of 1993, 48
Health Services Cost Review Commission (Maryland), 125
HealthStream Research, 84
HEDIS. *See* Healthcare Effectiveness Data and Information Set
Heifetz, Ronald, 8, 73, 109
Hermann Hospital (Texas): Memorial Hermann Physician Network's acquisition of, 87
Hidden agendas, 167
Hipp, Charlie, 71, 72, 73, 75, 76
Hippocrates, xix
Hippocratic oath, 102n2

Hiring: of primary care physicians at Salem Hospital, 109; at Stillwater Medical Group, 75–76; ThedaCare compact and, 63–64; Virginia Mason Medical Center compact and, 34

Hoffman, R., xx

Holloway, David, 106, 107, 110, 111, 112, 113, 114, 116, 122

Hospital boards, 105, 150

Hospitals & Health Networks magazine, 63

Hospitalist program: for ThedaCare, 51

HSCRC. *See* Health Services Cost Review Commission

HSS. *See* US Department of Health and Human Services

Human resources policies and procedures: implementation of compact and, 162–63

Human resources practices: building new, 154

ICSI. *See* Institute for Clinical Systems Improvement

Idealized Design of Clinical Office Practices (IDCOP) collaborative, 50

IHI. *See* Institute for Healthcare Improvement

Implicit reciprocal agreements, xix

Independent physician associations, 83, 84, 85

Individual autonomy: professional autonomy *vs.,* 121

Informed Medical Decisions Foundation, 78

Institute for Clinical Systems Improvement (Minneapolis), 71, 72, 82

Institute for Healthcare Improvement, 11, 24, 50; Annual Forum workshops, 111; "Boards on Board" initiative, 106, 107, 110; Triple Aim, 123

Institute of Medicine, 22

Internal staff: competent, 151

IPAs. *See* Independent physician associations

Jacobs, Andrew, 31, 33, 34, 39

JCC. *See* Joint conference committee

Job descriptions: compact implementation and, 162

Job security: loyalty and, xix–xx

JOC. *See* Joint operating committee

Johnson, Marty, 121, 122

Join the Club: How Peer Pressure Can Change the World (Rosenberg), 102n2

Joint conference committee: at Salem Hospital, 111, 112

Joint operating committee: at Memorial Hermann Physician Network, 95

Kaissi, Amer, 4

kaizen: ThedaCare and, 52; Virginia Mason Medical Center and, 19, 32

kaizen in boardroom of Virginia Mason Medical Center, 41–44; assets of hiring from outside, 43–44; board compact and transformation at Virginia Mason, 41–42; board compact development, 42; compact as document of real value, 44; headings from board compact, *43;* new roles for board membership, 42; understanding the need for change, 42; using the compact, 43

Kaplan, Gary, 19, 20, 27, 28, 29, 30, 31, 32, 33, 45, 129; elected as CEO, at Virginia Mason Medical Center, 23–24; Japanese study tour organized by, 42; leadership compact and, 39; on life for new Virginia Mason doctors, 20; physician and leadership recruitment and, 34; September 2000 retreat and, 24, 25–27; on unarticulated board compact, 41–42

Kenney, Charles, 20

Kim, W. Chan, 55

Kimberly-Clark Corporation, 49

Kotter, John, 31

Kramer, Dawna, 27

Lakeview Health System (Minnesota), 80; merger with HealthPartners, 82

Lakeview Hospital (Minnesota), 69, 70, 73

Lammert, Joyce, 24, 25, 27, 28, 29, 33, 36

LCQ. *See* Leading a Culture of Quality

Leaders: as active participants, 150; with clear purpose, 150; compact implementation and actions of, 163; as sponsors and visible supporters, 149–51

Leadership compact: at Virginia Mason Medical Center, 38, 39–41, *40,* 176–77

Memorial Hermann Physician Network
(*continued*)
   hardwiring physician influence in decision making in, *99*; summary of success factors in, *99*–101; "up and over" mechanism and, 95–96; weaknesses recognized in, 86; widely dispersed, independent-minded physicians in, 83–84
Memorial Hermann Southwest Hospital (Texas), 88
MHHNP. *See* Memorial Hermann Health Network Providers
MHHS. *See* Memorial Hermann Health System
MHMD. *See* Memorial Hermann Physician Network
Miller, Diane, 24, 39, 40
Mireles, Leticia, 94
Morrissey, Larry, 72, 74, 75, 77, 78, 79, 82
MPRC. *See* Multispecialty peer-review committee
Multisite organizations: Silversin on compacts for, 168–69
Multispecialty peer-review committee: at Salem Hospital, 116, 119
Mutual expectations: clarifying, 166

Nagele-Vitalis, Carol, 73
Nakao, Chihiro, 31
Naleppa, Peggy, 130, 132, 133, 136, 138, 139
Nance, John, 25
National Committee for Quality Assurance, 50
National Health Service (England), 141; Trust Development Authority, 142
NCQA. *See* National Committee for Quality Assurance
Negative judgments: as dead ends for compact process, 151–52
New-world compact: summary of, xx
NHS. *See* National Health Service
Norton, Claire, 120
Novus Health Group. *See* ThedaCare Physicians
Nurse practitioners (NPs): Silversin on compacts and, 170
Nurses: Virginia Mason's physician compact and, 38

Ohno, Taiichi, 31
On-boarding: implementation of compact and, 162
On the Mend (Toussaint and Gerard), 52
Organization: Silversin on accountability, compacts, and, 171–72
Organizational imperatives: mismatch between physician expectations and, 6, *7*
Organization Man, The (Whyte), xix
Orlikoff, Jamie, 44
Outreach: compact implementation and, 162
Oversight: sustained results and, 155–56

PAs. *See* Physician assistants
Patient care: physician engagement and compacts speaking to, 153
Patient-centered care: at Stillwater Medical Group, 77, *81*; at Virginia Mason Medical Center, 19–20, 22, 39
Patterson, Sarah, 40
PDSA cycle. *See* Plan-do-study-act cycle
PEC. *See* Physician Excellence Committee
Peer-review problem: at Peninsula Regional Medical Center, 128
Peer-review process: revamped, at Salem Hospital, 116, 119
Peninsula Regional Medical Center (Maryland), xxii, 125–40, 153; background, 126; compact approval at, 133; compact for, sample tenets, *134*; compact work back on track at, 137; drafting committee at, 131–33; evolution in hospital at, 136–37; evolution in medical staff at, 135–36; former, unspoken compact at, 126–27; increasing synchronicity at, 134–37; location of, 125; medical staff leaders push for new compact at, 127–30; ongoing challenges at, 138–39; peer-review problem at, 128; Physician Compact, 189; reimbursement problem at, 128–29; retreat and call to action for, 130–31; summary of compact work at, 139–40
Pensions: ThedaCare, top-down changes, and, 53
Perceptions activity: trust and, 167
Performance: compact implementation and, 15, 162

Protection, xviii, 22; newer generation of physicians and, xxi; physicians' tacit expectations of, 6, *7*; Salem Hospital physicians and, 108

Provider inclusion: Silversin on compacts and, 170

Psychological contract, 108; definition of, 4–5; origins of, xix–xx

Psychological safety: skilled facilitators and, 148–49

QOC. *See* Quality operations committee

Qualheim, Kathy, 55

Qualified clinically integrated joint arrangements: criteria for, 85

Quality-improvement movement: compact dialogue and, 11

Quality measures: publicly reported, Stillwater Medical Group and, 78

Quality operations committee: at Salem Hospital, 119–20

Ratification of compact, 14–15

Reciprocal accountability: embedding mechanisms for, 154–55

Reciprocity of commitments: draft compact and, 160–61

Recognition programs: compact implementation and, 162–63

Recruitment: implementation of compact and, 162

Reform. *See* Healthcare reform

Reimbursement: at Peninsula Regional Medical Center, 128–29

Reinertsen, J. L., 120, 132, 139

Relationships: improving, compact creation and, 148–49

Rensel, Kimberly, 89

Representation: multisite organizations and, 169

Rewards: compact implementation and, 162–63

Riccio, Thomas J., 125, 127, 128, 129, 130, 131, 132, 133, 136, 138

Rona, Mike, 26

Rosenberg, Tina, 102n2

Rousseau, Denise, 4

Sabotage, 167

Salem Clinic (Oregon): compact at, 117–19; Physician Compact, 188

Salem Hospital (Oregon), xxii, 103–23; adaptive changes hard to accept and risky to lead at, 109; board input at, 113–14; building common ground at, 110–12; challenges in moving beyond "good enough" at, 106–9; Common Ground Compact, *115,* 186–87; compact as keystone at, 116, 119–21; compact implementation committee at, 114–16; drafting compact for, 113; employing physicians exacerbates tensions at, 108–9; executive leadership issues in, 105–6; expanding leadership at, 113; four-part development program at, 151; hospital–doctor relationship and, 104–5; inadequate physician accountability at, 108; location of, 103; new chief medical officer who relates to physicians, 106–7; patient-oriented building program for, 107; realization that shared vision was needed for, 110–11; shared vision defined for, 112–13; skepticism of administration's motives at, 107–8; summary of experiences at, 123; taking on compact work at, 111–12; tensions escalate at, 104–6; unfinished journey at, 122

Scallon, Steve, 69, 70, 75

Schein, Edgar: on psychological contract, xix

Schembre, Drew, 27

Scott, Pat, 27

"See, feel, change" process: meaningful change and, 31

Senge, Peter, xxii

Servant leadership: at ThedaCare, 60

Service line co-management: at Peninsula Regional Medical Center, 137

SHA. *See* Strategic Health Authority

Shabot, Michael, 88, 90, 95

Shared vision, 160

Sherman, Ken, 113, 115

Silversin, Jack, xxii, 11, 103, 141, 150; Institute for Clinical Systems Improvement collaborative and, 72; Memorial Hermann Physician Network

About the Author and Collaborator

Mary Jane Kornacki and **Jack Silversin** are the founding partners of Amicus, a healthcare consulting firm based in Cambridge, Massachusetts. Their breakthrough work on physician compacts is helping organizations to achieve better results from change efforts and to improve physician morale and commitment.

Mary Jane holds a master of science degree in public health from the University of Massachusetts, where she specialized in health education and health behavior. Her professional interests include leadership, team dynamics, and organizational culture and professional subcultures within medical organizations. Her understanding of the principles of adult learning and behavior change is reflected in the models and tools that are fundamental to the pair's consulting work and to this book. She has developed, and trained facilitators to deliver, programs on improving patient relations and strengthening healthcare team dynamics.

A graduate of the Harvard University School of Dental Medicine and a member of its Faculty of Medicine, Jack holds a doctorate in public health from Harvard University. He is Institute for Healthcare Improvement faculty and presents regularly at its national and international conferences. His clients include many successful, innovative community and academic healthcare organizations and systems across the United States.

The pair have collaborated on numerous publications on physician cultures, physician morale, medical group dynamics, governance in physician organizations, and service improvement in healthcare. They also coauthored *Leading Physicians Through Change: How to Achieve and Sustain Results,* second edition, American College of Physician Executives, 2012.

You can learn more about their work at their website, www.consultamicus.com.